Mosby's

PHYSICAL EXAMINATION HANDBOOK

Mosby's
PHYSICAL EXAMINATION HANDBOOK

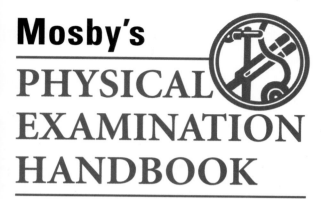

HENRY M. SEIDEL, MD
Professor Emeritus of Pediatrics
School of Medicine
The Johns Hopkins University
Baltimore, Maryland

JANE W. BALL, RN, DrPH, CPNP
Director, Emergency Medical Services for Children
National Resource Center
Children's National Medical Center
Washington, DC

JOYCE E. DAINS, DrPH, JD, RN, CS, FNP
Assistant Professor
Baylor College of Medicine
Houston, Texas

G. WILLIAM BENEDICT, MD, PhD
Assistant Professor, Medicine
School of Medicine
The Johns Hopkins University
Baltimore, Maryland

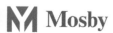 Mosby

A Harcourt Health Sciences Company

St. Louis   London   Philadelphia   Sydney   Toronto

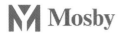

A Harcourt Health Sciences Company

SECOND EDITION

Copyright © 1999 by Mosby, Inc.

Previous edition copyrighted 1995.

Compostion by Graphic World Inc.

Mosby, Inc.
11830 Westline Industrial Drive
St. Louis, Missouri 63146

Library of Congress Cataloging-in-Publication Data
Mosby's physical examination handbook / Henry M. Seidel . . . [et al.].
  —2nd ed.
    p.   cm.
  Includes bibliographical references and index.
  ISBN 0-323-00179-3
  1. Physical diagnosis—Handbooks, manuals, etc.   I. Seidel, Henry M.
  [DNLM: 1. Physical Examination—methods handbook.   WB 39M894 1999]
  RC76.M64   1999
  616.07′54—dc21
  DNLM/DLC   98-27273

00 01 02 / 9 8 7 6 5 4 3 2

Contents

Pediatric Variations

INTRODUCTION

Mosby's Physical Examination Handbook is a portable clinical reference on physical examination that is suitable for students of nursing, medicine, chiropractic, and other allied health disciplines, as well as for practicing health care providers. It offers brief descriptions of examination techniques and guidelines on how the examination should proceed step by step. This text is intended to be an aid to review and recall the procedures for physical examination.

The text begins with an outline of what information should be obtained for the patient's medical history and gives a brief review of the body systems. The next two chapters address assessment of the patient's mental status and nutritional status. Subsequent chapters for each of the body systems list equipment needed to perform the examination and present the techniques to be used. Expected and unexpected findings follow the description of each technique. More than 196 full color illustrations interspersed throughout the text reinforce recall of techniques and possible findings. Each chapter offers aids to differential diagnosis and also provides sample documentation.

A new feature of this edition is a section at the end of each chapter that details variations for pediatric patients. These sections are highlighted by a colored screen to make access to the information easy when you are conducting a pediatric examination. A new chapter that outlines variations of the head-to-toe examination in regard to specific age-groups of pediatric patients and a chapter that outlines what to include in a "well-woman examination" have also been added.

Chapter 18 gives an overview of the complete examination, and Chapter 21 gives guidelines for reporting and recording information gathered in the examination.

CHAPTER 1

The History

TAKING THE HISTORY

The following outline of what to include when taking a patient history should be viewed not as a rigid structure but a general guideline. Since you are beginning your relationship with the patient at this point, pay attention to this relationship as well as to the information you seek in the history. Be friendly and show respect for the patient. Choose a comfortable setting and help the patient get settled. Maintain eye contact and use a conversational tone. Begin by introducing yourself and explaining your role. Help the patient understand why you are taking the history and how it will be used. Once the history proceeds, explore positive responses with additional questions: where, when, what, how, and why. Be sensitive to the patient's emotions at all times.

CHIEF COMPLAINT

The problem or symptom: reason for visit
Duration of problem
Patient information: age, sex, marital status; previous hospital admissions; occupation
Other complaints: secondary issues, fears, concerns; what made the patient seek care

PRESENT PROBLEM

Chronologic ordering: sequence of events patient has experienced
State of health just before the onset of the present problem
Complete description of the first symptom: time and date of onset, location, movement
Possible exposure to infection or toxic agents
If symptoms intermittent, describe typical attack: onset, duration, symptoms, variations, inciting factors, exacerbating factors, relieving factors

Impact of illness: on life-style, on ability to function, limitations imposed by illness

"Stability" of the problem: intensity, variations, improvement, worsening, staying the same

Immediate reason for seeking attention, particularly for long-standing problem

Review of appropriate system when there is a conspicuous disturbance of a particular organ or system

Medications: current and recent, dosage of prescriptions, home remedies, nonprescription medications

Review of chronology of events for each problem: patient's confirmations and corrections.

MEDICAL HISTORY

General health and strength

Childhood illnesses: measles, mumps, whooping cough, chicken pox, smallpox, scarlet fever, acute rheumatic fever, diphtheria, poliomyelitis

Major adult illnesses: tuberculosis (TB), hepatitis, diabetes, hypertension, myocardial infarction, tropical or parasitic diseases, other infections, any nonsurgical hospital admissions

Immunizations: poliomyelitis, diphtheria, pertussis, and tetanus toxoid, influenza, cholera, typhus, typhoid, bacille Calmette-Guérin (BCG), hepatitis B virus (HBV), last purified protein derivative (PPD) or other skin tests; unusual reactions to immunizations; tetanus or other antitoxin made with horse serum

Surgery: dates, hospital, diagnosis, complications

Serious injuries: resulting disability (document fully for injuries with possible legal implications)

Limitation of ability to function as desired as a result of past events

Medications, past, current, and recent medications; dosage of prescription; home remedies and nonprescription medications

Allergies: especially to medications, but also to environmental allergens and foods

Transfusions: reactions, date, and number of units transfused

Emotional status: mood disorders, psychiatric treatment

Children: birth, developmental milestones, childhood diseases, immunizations

FAMILY HISTORY

Relatives with similar illness

Immediate family: ethnicity, health, cause of and age at death

History of disease: heart disease, high blood pressure, hypercholesterolemia, cancer, TB, stroke, epilepsy, diabetes, gout, kidney disease, thyroid disease, asthma and other allergic states; forms of arthritis; blood diseases; sexually transmitted diseases; other familial diseases

Spouse and children: age, health

Hereditary disease: history of grandparents, aunts, uncles, siblings, cousins, consanguinity

PERSONAL AND SOCIAL HISTORY

Personal status: birthplace, where raised; home environment; parental divorce or separation, socioeconomic class, cultural background; education; position in family; marital status; general life satisfaction; hobbies and interests; sources of stress and strain

Habits: nutrition and diet, regularity and patterns of eating and sleeping; exercise: quantity and type; quantity of coffee, tea, tobacco; alcohol; illicit drugs: frequency, type, amount; breast or testicular self-examination

Sexual history: concerns with sexual feelings and performance; frequency of intercourse, ability to achieve orgasm, number and variety of partners

Home conditions: housing, economic condition, type of health insurance if any; pets and their health

Occupation: description of usual work and present work if different; list of job changes; work conditions and hours; physical and mental strain; duration of employment; present and past exposure to heat and cold, industrial toxins, especially lead, arsenic, chromium, asbestos, beryllium, poisonous gases, benzene, and polyvinyl chloride or other carcinogens and teratogens; any protective devices required, for example, goggles or masks

Environment: travel and other exposure to contagious diseases, residence in tropics, water and milk supply, other sources of infection if applicable

Military record: dates and geographic area of assignments

Religious preference: determine any religious proscriptions concerning medical care

Cost of care: resources available to patient, financial worries, candid discussion of issues

REVIEW OF SYSTEMS

General constitutional symptoms: fever, chills, malaise, fatigability, night sweats; weight (average, preferred, present, change)

Diet: appetite, likes and dislikes, restrictions (because of religion, allergy, or disease), vitamins and other supplements, use of caffeine-containing beverages (coffee, tea, cola); an hour-by-hour detailing of food and liquid intake—sometimes a written diary covering several days of intake may be necessary

Skin, hair, and nails: rash or eruption, itching, pigmentation or texture change; excessive sweating, abnormal nail or hair growth

Musculoskeletal: joint stiffness, pain, restriction of motion, swelling, redness, heat, bony deformity

Head and neck:

General: frequent or unusual headaches, their location, dizziness, syncope, severe head injuries; periods of loss of consciousness (momentary or prolonged)

Eyes: visual acuity, blurring, diplopia, photophobia, pain, recent change in appearance or vision; glaucoma, use of eye drops or other eye medications; history of trauma or familial eye disease

Ears: hearing loss, pain, discharge, tinnitus, vertigo

Nose: sense of smell, frequency of colds, obstruction, epistaxis, postnasal discharge, sinus pain

Throat and mouth: hoarseness or change in voice; frequent sore throats, bleeding or swelling of gums; recent tooth abscesses or extractions; soreness of tongue or buccal mucosa, ulcers; disturbance of taste

Endocrine thyroid enlargement or tenderness, heat or cold intolerance, unexplained weight change, diabetes, polydipsia, polyuria, changes in facial or body hair, increased hat and glove size, skin striae

Males: puberty onset, erections, emissions, testicular pain, libido, infertility

Females:

Menses: onset, regularity, duration and amount of flow, dysmenorrhea, last period, intermenstrual discharge or bleeding, itching, date of last Pap smear, age at menopause, libido, frequency of intercourse, sexual difficulties, infertility

Pregnancies: number, miscarriages, abortions, duration of pregnancy, each type of delivery, any complications during any pregnancy or postpartum period or with neonate, use of oral or other contraceptives

Breasts: pain, tenderness, discharge, lumps, galactorrhea, mammograms (screening or diagnostic), frequency of breast self-examination

Chest and lungs: pain related to respiration, dyspnea, cyanosis, wheezing, cough, sputum (character and quantity), hemoptysis, night sweats, exposure to TB; date and result of last chest x-ray examination

Heart and blood vessels: chest pain or distress, precipitating causes, timing and duration, character; relieving factors; palpitations, dyspnea, orthopnea (number of pillows needed), edema, claudication, hypertension, previous myocardial infarction, estimate of exercise tolerance, past electrocardiogram (ECG) or other cardiac tests

Hematologic: anemia, tendency to bruise or bleed easily, thromboses, thrombophlebitis, any known abnormality of blood cells, transfusions

Lymph nodes: enlargement, tenderness, suppuration

Gastrointestinal: appetite, digestion, intolerance for any class of foods, dysphagia, heartburn, nausea, vomiting, hematemesis, regularity of bowels, constipation, diarrhea, change in stool color or contents (clay-colored, tarry, fresh blood, mucus, undigested food), flatulence, hemorrhoids, hepatitis, jaundice, dark urine, history of ulcer, gallstones, polyps, tumor; previous x-ray examinations (where, when, findings)

Genitourinary: dysuria, flank or suprapubic pain, urgency, frequency, nocturia, hematuria, polyuria, hesitancy, dribbling, loss in force of stream, passage of stone; edema of face, stress incontinence, hernias, sexually transmitted disease (inquire type and symptoms, and results of serologic test for syphilis, if known)

Neurologic: syncope, seizures, weakness or paralysis, abnormalities of sensation or coordination, tremors, loss of memory

Psychiatric: depression, mood changes, difficulty concentrating, nervousness, tension, suicidal thoughts, irritability, sleep disturbances

Taking the history

These are only guidelines; you are free to modify and add as the needs of your patients and your judgment may dictate.

Chief complaint

A parent or other responsible adult will generally be the major resource. Still, when age permits, the child should be involved as much as possible. Remember, too, that every chief complaint has the potential of an underlying concern. What is it that really led to the visit to you? Was it just the sore throat?

Reliability

Note the relationship to the patient of the person who is the resource for the history and record your impression of the competence of that person as a historian.

Present problem

Be sure to give a clear chronologic sequence to the story.

Medical history

In general, the age of the patient and/or the nature of the problem will guide your approach to the history. Clearly, in a continuing relationship much of what is to be known will already have been recorded. Certainly, different aspects of the past history require varying emphasis depending on the nature of the immediate problem. There are specifics that will command attention.

Pregnancy/mother's health:
   Infectious disease; give approximate gestational month
   Weight gain/edema
   Hypertension
   Proteinuria
   Bleeding; approximate time
   Eclampsia; threat of eclampsia
   Special or unusual diet or dietary practices
   Medications (hormones, vitamins)
   Quality of fetal movements; time of onset
   Radiation exposure
   Prenatal care/consistency
Birth and the perinatal experience:

Duration of pregnancy

Delivery site

Labor: spontaneous/induced; duration; anesthesia; complications

Delivery: presentation; forceps/spontaneous; complications

Condition at birth: time of onset of cry; Apgar scores, if available

Birth weight and, if available, length and head circumference

Neonatal period:

Hospital experience: length of stay, feeding experience, oxygen needs, vigor, color (jaundice, cyanosis), cry. Did baby go home with mother?

First month of life: color (jaundice), feeding, vigor; any suggestion of illness or untoward event

Feeding:

Bottle or breast: any changes and why; type of formula: amounts offered, taken; frequency; weight gain

Present diet and appetite; introduction of solids, current routine and frequency, age weaned from bottle or breast, daily intake of milk, food preferences, ability to feed self; elaborate on any feeding problems

Development

The guidelines suggested in Chapter 20, Head-to-Toe Examination: Infants, Children, and Adolescents, are complementary to the milestones listed below. Those included here are commonly used, often remembered, and often recorded in "baby books." Photographs may also be of some help occasionally.

Age when

Held head erect while held in sitting position

Sat alone, unsupported

Walked alone

Talked in sentences

Toilet trained

School: grade, performance, learning and social problems

Dentition: ages for first teeth, loss of deciduous teeth, and first permanent teeth

Growth: height and weight at different ages, changes in rate of growth or weight gain or loss

Sexual: present status, e.g., in female, time of breast development, nipples, pubic hair, description of menses; in males, development of pubic hair, voice change, acne, emissions. Follow Tanner guides.

Family history

Maternal gestational history, all pregnancies with status of each, including date, age, and cause of death of all deceased siblings, and dates and duration of pregnancy in the case of miscarriages; mother's health during pregnancy

Age of parents at birth of patient

Are the parents related in any way?

Personal and social history

Personal status:
   School adjustment
   Nail biting
   Thumb sucking
   Breath holding
   Temper tantrums
   Pica
   Tics
   Rituals
Home conditions:
   Parent(s)' occupation(s)
   Principal caretaker(s) of the patient
   Food preparation, routine, family preferences (e.g., vegetarianism), who does the preparing
   Adequacy of clothing
   Dependency on relief or social agencies
   Number of persons and rooms in the house or apartment
   Sleeping routines and sleep arrangements for the child

Review of systems (some suggested additional questions or particular concerns)

Ears: otitis media (frequency, laterality)
Nose: snoring, mouth breathing
Teeth: dental care
Genitourinary: nature of the urinary stream, forceful or a dribble
Skin, hair, and nails: eczema or seborrhea

CHAPTER 2

Mental Status

EQUIPMENT

- Familiar objects (coins, keys, paper clips)
- Paper and pencil

EXAMINATION

Perform the mental status examination throughout the entire patient interaction. Focus on the individual's strengths and capabilities for executive functioning (motivation, initiative, goal formation, planning and performing work or activities, self-monitoring, and integration of feedback from various sources to refine or redirect energy). Interview a family member or friend if you have any concerns about the patient's responses or behaviors.

Use a mental status screening examination for health visits when no cognitive, emotional, or behavior problems are apparent. Information is generally observed during the history in the following areas:

Appearance and Behavior
    Grooming
    Emotional status
    Body language

Emotional stability
    Mood and feelings
    Thought process and content

Cognitive abilities
    State of consciousness
    Memory
    Attention span
    Judgment

Speech and language
    Voice quality
    Articulation
    Comprehension
    Coherence
    Ability to communicate

TECHNIQUE	FINDINGS

Mental Status and Speech Patterns

Observe physical appearance and behavior

- *Grooming*

  UNEXPECTED: Poor hygiene, lack of concern with appearance, or inappropriate dress for season, gender, or occasion in previously well-groomed patient.

- *Emotional status*

  EXPECTED: Patient expressing concern with visit appropriate for emotional content of topics discussed.

  UNEXPECTED: Behavior conveying carelessness, indifference, inability to sense emotions in others, loss of sympathetic reactions, unusual docility, rage reactions, agitation, or excessive irritability.

- *Body language*

  EXPECTED: Erect posture and eye contact (if culturally appropriate).

  UNEXPECTED: Slumped posture, lack of facial expression, inappropriate affect, excessively energetic movements, or constantly watchful eyes.

Investigate cognitive abilities

- *The Mini-Mental State Examination*
  Use this examination to quantify cognitive function or document changes (See pp. 12-13.)

  EXPECTED: Score of 21-30.

  UNEXPECTED: Score of 20 or less. Significant memory loss, confusion, impaired communication.

- *State of consciousness*

  EXPECTED: Oriented to time, place, and person, and able to appropriately respond to questions and environmental stimuli.

TECHNIQUE	FINDINGS

UNEXPECTED: Disorientation to time, place, or person. Verbal response is confused, incoherent or inappropriate, or no verbal response.

- *The Set Test*
Use this test to evaluate mental status as a whole (motivation, alertness, concentration, short-term memory, problem solving). Ask the patient to name 10 items in each of 4 groups: fruit, animals, colors, and town/cities. Give each item 1 point for a maximum of 40 points.

EXPECTED: Able to categorize, count, and remember items listed. Score of 25 or more points.

UNEXPECTED: Score less than 15 points. Check for mental changes or cultural, educational, or social factors when score is 15 to 24.

- *Analogies*
Ask patient to describe analogies, first simple, then more complex:
  · What is similar about peaches and lemons, oceans and lakes, pencils and typewriters?
  · An engine is to an airplane as an oar is to a _____?
  · What is different about a magazine and a telephone book, and bush and tree?

UNEXPECTED: Inability to describe similarities or differences.

- *Abstract reasoning*
Ask patient to explain meaning of fable, proverb, or metaphor:
  · A stich in time saves nine.
  · A bird in the hand is worth two in the bush.

UNEXPECTED: Inability to give adequate explanation.

Patient ....
Examiner ....
Date ....

MINI-MENTAL STATE EXAMINATION

Maximum Score	Score	
		ORIENTATION
5	( )	What is the (year) (season) (date) (day) (month)?
5	( )	Where are we: (state) (county) (town) (hospital) (floor)?
		REGISTRATION
3	( )	Name 3 objects: 1 second to say each. Then ask the patient all 3 after you have said them. Give 1 point for each correct answer. Then repeat them until he learns all 3. Count trials and record. #Trials _____
		ATTENTION AND CALCULATION
5	( )	Serial 7's. 1 point for each correct. Stop after 5 answers. Alternatively spell "world" backwards.
		RECALL
3	( )	Ask for the 3 objects repeated above. Give 1 point for each correct.
		LANGUAGE
9	( )	Name a pencil, and watch (2 points)
		Repeat the following "No ifs, ands, or buts." (1 point)
		Follow a 3-stage command:
		"Take a paper in your right hand, fold it in half, and put it on the floor" (3 points)
		Read and obey the following: CLOSE YOUR EYES (1 point)
		Write a sentence (1 point)
		Copy design (1 point)
___		Total score
		ASSESS level of consciousness along a continuum _____

Alert   Drowsy   Stupor   Coma

INSTRUCTIONS FOR ADMINISTRATION OF MINI-MENTAL STATE EXAMINATION

ORIENTATION

(1) Ask for the date. Then ask specifically for parts omitted, e.g., "Can you also tell me what season it is?" One point for each correct.

(2) Ask in turn "Can you tell me the name of this hospital?" (town, county, etc.). One point for each correct.

REGISTRATION

Ask the patient if you may test his memory. Then say the name of 3 unrelated objects, clearly and slowly, about one second for each. After you have said 3, ask him to repeat them. The first repetition determines his score (0-3) but keep saying them until he can repeat all 3, up to 6 trials. If he does not eventually learn all 3, recall cannot be meaningfully tested.

ATTENTION AND CALCULATION

Ask the patient to begin with 100 and count backwards by 7. Stop after 5 subtractions (93, 86, 79, 72, 65). Score the total number of correct answers.

If the patient cannot or will not perform this task, ask him to spell the word "world" backwards. The score is the number of letters in correct order.
E.g. dlrow = 5, dlorw = 3.

RECALL

Ask the patient if he can recall the 3 words you previously asked him to remember. Score 0-3.

LANGUAGE

Naming: Show the patient a wrist watch and ask him what it is. Repeat for pencil. Score 0-2.

Repetition: Ask the patient to repeat the sentence after you. Allow only one trial. Score 0 or 1.

3-Stage command: Give the patient a piece of plain blank paper and repeat the command. Score 1 point for each part correctly executed.

Reading: On a blank piece of paper print the sentence "Close your eyes," in letters large enough for the patient to see clearly. Ask him to read it and do what it says. Score 1 point only if he actually closes his eyes.

Writing: Give the patient a blank piece of paper and ask him to write a sentence for you. Do not dictate a sentence; it is to be written spontaneously. It must contain a subject and verb and be sensible. Correct grammar and punctuation are not necessary.

Copying: On a clean piece of paper, draw intersecting pentagons, each side about 1 in., and ask him to copy it exactly as it is. All 10 angles must be present and 2 must intersect to score 1 point. Tremor and rotation are ignored.

Estimate the patient's level of sensorium along a continuum, from alert on the left to coma on the right.

From Folstein et al, 1985.

TECHNIQUE	FINDINGS

- A rolling stone gathers no moss.

■ *Arithmetic calculations*
Ask patient to perform simple calculations without paper:
  - 50 − 7, −7, −7, etc., until the answer is 8.
  - 50 + 8, +8. +8. etc., until the answer is 98.

UNEXPECTED: Inability to complete with few errors within a minute.

■ *Writing ability*
Ask patient to write name and address or a phrase you dictate (or draw simple figures—triangle, circle, square, flower, house—if unable to write).

UNEXPECTED: Omission or addition of letters, syllables, or words; mirror writing; or uncoordinated writing (or drawing for patients unable to write).

■ *Execution of motor skills*
Ask patient to do a motor task such as combing hair.

UNEXPECTED: Inability to complete a task.

■ *Memory*
Immediate recall: Ask patient to listen to, then repeat, a sentence or series of numbers (5 to 8 numbers forward, 4 to 6 numbers backward).
Recent memory: Show patient four or five objects or give the visually impaired patient four unrelated words with distinct sounds to remember (carpet, iris, bench, fortune). Say you will ask about them later. In 10 minutes, ask patient to list objects.

EXPECTED: Immediate recall: Able to repeat sentence or numbers.
Recent memory: Able to remember test objects.
Remote memory: Able to recall verifiable past events.
UNEXPECTED: Impaired memory. Loss of immediate and recent memory with retention of remote memory.

TECHNIQUE	FINDINGS

Remote memory: Ask patient about verifiable past events (e.g., mother's maiden name, name of high school).

■ *Attention span*
Ask the patient to follow a series of short commands (e.g., take off all clothes, put on patient gown, and sit on examining table).

EXPECTED: Responds to directions appropriately.
UNEXPECTED: Easy distraction or confusion, negativism.

■ *Judgment*
Explore:
· How patient meets social and family obligations; patient's future plans.
· Patient's solutions to hypothetical situations (e.g., found stamped envelope or was stopped for running red light).

EXPECTED: Ability to evaluate situation and provide appropriate response; managing business affairs appropriately.
UNEXPECTED: Response indicating hazardous behavior or inappropriate action.

Evaluate emotional stability

■ *Mood and feelings*
Ask patient how he or she feels, if feelings are a problem in daily life, and if he or she has particularly difficult times or experiences.

EXPECTED: Appropriate feelings for the situation.
UNEXPECTED: Unresponsiveness, hopelessness, agitation, euphoria, irritablility, or wide mood swings.

■ *Thought process and content*
· Ask patient about obsessive thoughts and compulsive behavior
· Observe sequence, logic, coherence, and relevance of topics.

EXPECTED: Appropriate sequence, logic, coherence, and relevance to topics discussed.
UNEXPECTED: Illogical or unrealistic thought process, blocking, or disturbance in stream of thinking. Obsessive thought content or behavior that interferes with daily life or is disabling.

TECHNIQUE	FINDINGS

■ *Perceptual distortions and hallucinations*
Ask patient about any sensations not believed caused by external stimuli. Find out when these experiences occur.

UNEXPECTED: Auditory, visual, or tactile hallucinations: hears voices, sees vivid images or shadowy figures, smells offensive odors, feels worms crawling on skin.

Observe speech and language

■ *Voice quality*

EXPECTED: Patient uses inflections, speaks clearly and strongly, and is able to increase voice volume and pitch.
UNEXPECTED: Difficulty or discomfort making laryngeal speech sounds or varying volume, quality, or pitch of speech.

■ *Articulation*

EXPECTED: Proper pronunciation, fluent, and rhythmic, easily expresses thoughts.
UNEXPECTED: Imperfect pronunciation, difficulty articulating single speech sound, rapid-fire delivery, or speech with hesitancy, stuttering, repetitions, or slow utterances.

■ *Comprehension*

EXPECTED: Able to follow simple instructions.

■ *Coherence*

EXPECTED: Patient's intentions or perceptions clearly conveyed.
UNEXPECTED: Circumlocutions, perseveration, flight of ideas or loosening of associations between thoughts, gibberish, neologisms, echolalia, or unusual sounds.

TECHNIQUE	FINDINGS
■ *Ability to communicate*	**UNEXPECTED:** Hesitations, omissions, inappropriate word substitutions, circumlocutions, neologisms, disturbance of rhythm or words in sequence or other signs of aphasia.

AIDS TO DIFFERENTIAL DIAGNOSIS

ABNORMALITY	DESCRIPTION
Depression	Mood and affect include extreme sadness, anxiety, and irritability. Lack of motivation, lethargic or restless and agitated. Inability to concentrate.
Dementia	Insidious onset; depressed, apathetic mood persists. Rambling or incoherent speech. Memory, judgment, thought patterns, and calculations impaired. Progressive condition.
Delirium	Sudden onset; this condition lasts for hours or days. Mood and affect include rapid mood swings, fear, and suspicion. Slurred or rapid and manic speech and hallucinations are common. Sleep-wake cycle may be disturbed.
Dementia of Alzheimer's type	Subtle onset—generally with early memory loss, impaired ability to learn new information, or disturbance in executive functioning—leading to profound disintegration of personality and complete disorientation. Varied duration and rate of progression.

ABNORMALITY	DESCRIPTION
Mental retardation	Subaverage intellectual functioning, deficits in adaptive behavior, inability to discriminate among stimuli, impaired short-term memory, lack of motivation.

PEDIATRIC VARIATIONS

EXAMINATION

TECHNIQUE	FINDINGS

Mental Status

Use the parent's impressions of the infant's responsiveness to guide your assessment.

EXPECTED: Infant responds appropriately to parent's voice—is attentive, comforts easily.

Child follows simple directions, performs age-appropriate skills (Chapter 20).

UNEXPECTED: Nonresponsive, inconsolable, combative, lethargic.

AIDS TO DIFFERENTIAL DIAGNOSIS

ABNORMALITY	DESCRIPTION
Autistic disorder	Development disorder with odd repetitive behaviors, preoccupation with objects, an aversion to touch, delayed language or echolalia. Motor development may progress as expected.

Mental status. Appropriate dress and behavior. Oriented to time, place, and person. Reasoning and arithmetic calculations abilities intact. Immediate, recent, and remote memory intact. Appropriate mood and feeling expressed. Speech clearly and smoothly enunciated; comprehends directions.

CLINICAL AND
REFERENCE NOTES

CHAPTER 3

Nutrition and Growth and Measurement

EQUIPMENT

- Tape measure with millimeter markings
- Calculator
- Skinfold caliper

EXAMINATION

TECHNIQUE	FINDINGS

Anthropometrics

Measure height and weight

Estimate desirable body weight (DBW)
Women: 100 lb for first 5 ft; plus 5 lb for each inch thereafter

EXPECTED: Add 10% for large frame; subtract 10% for small frame.

Men: 106 lb for first 5 ft; plus 6 lb for each inch thereafter

Use growth charts for pediatric patients, pp. 296-303.

Calculate % DBW

$$\frac{current\ weight}{DBW} \times 100$$

Calculate % usual body weight

$$\frac{current\ weight}{usual\ weight} \times 100$$

UNEXPECTED: Weight loss that equals or exceeds 1% to 2% in 1 week; 5% in 1 month; 7.5% in 3 months; 10% in 6 months.

Calculate % weight change

$$\frac{usual\ weight\ -\ current\ weight}{usual\ weight} \times 100$$

TECHNIQUE	FINDINGS

Calculate body mass index (BMI) (kg per m²)

$$\frac{\text{weight in lb} \times 705}{\text{height in inches}} \div$$

height in inches

or see nomogram below

EXPECTED: Women 19.1 to 27.3; men: 20.7 to 27.8.

UNEXPECTED: A BMI above 27.8 in men and 27.3 in women corresponds with being at least 20% overweight.

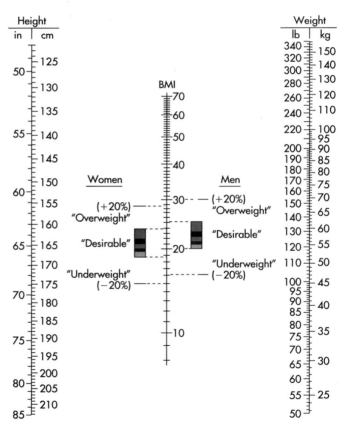

Nomogram for body mass index (kg/m/²). The weight/height² is read from the central scale. The ranges suggested as "desirable" are from life insurance data. *From Thomas AE et al, 1976.*

TECHNIQUE	FINDINGS

Calculate waist to hip circumference ratio

Using a tape measure with millimeter markings, measure the waist at or 1 cm above the umbilical midline. Then measure the hip at the level of the superior iliac crest. Divide the waist circumference by the hip circumference to obtain the ratio.

EXPECTED: Ratio less than 0.9 in men and 0.8 in women. **UNEXPECTED:** Ratios over 0.9 in men and 0.8 in women indicate increased risk of disease. This measurement has not been validated for use in the pediatric and adolescent populations.

Measure mid upper arm circumference (MAC)

Place tape around upper right arm, midway between the tips of the olecranon and acromial processes. Hold tape snugly and make the reading to the nearest 5 mm.

This measurement is obtained in order to calculate midarm muscle circumference (MAMC).

EXPECTED: 10% to 95%. **UNEXPECTED:** Less than 10%; greater than 95%. See the table below.

Percentiles for Arm Circumference, Midarm Muscle Circumference, and Triceps Skinfold

	MEN		WOMEN	
PERCENTILE	55-65 Y	65-75 Y	55-65 Y	65-75 Y
ARM CIRCUMFERENCE (CM)				
10th	27.3	26.3	25.7	25.2
50th	31.7	30.7	30.3	29.9
95th	36.9	35.5	38.5	37.3
ARM MUSCLE CIRCUMFERENCE (CM)				
10th	24.5	23.5	19.6	19.5
50th	27.8	26.8	22.5	22.5
95th	32.0	30.6	28.0	27.9
TRICEPS SKINFOLD (MM)				
10th	6	6	16	14
50th	11	11	25	24
95th	22	22	38	36

From Frisancho AR, 1981.

TECHNIQUE	FINDINGS

Measure triceps skinfold thickness (TSF)

Have the patient flex the right arm at a right angle. Find the midpoint between the tips of the olecranon and acromial process, and make a horizontal mark. Then draw a vertical line to intersect. With the arm relaxed, use your thumb and forefinger to grasp and lift the triceps skinfold about $1/_2$ inch proximal to the intersection marks. Place the caliper at the skinfold and measure. Make two readings and derive an average.

This measurement is obtained in order to calculate MAMC.

EXPECTED: 10% to 95%.
UNEXPECTED: Less than 10%; greater than 95%. See table on p. 23.

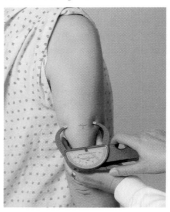

Calculate MAMC

MAMC = {MAC (mm) − [3.14 × TSF (mm)]}

EXPECTED: 10% to 95%.
UNEXPECTED: Less than 10%; greater than 95%. See table on p. 23.

Calculate estimates for energy needs

Use actual weight for healthy adults
Use adjusted weight for obese patients
Adjusted weight = [(actual body weight − DBW) × 25%] + DBW

CALORIES	KCAL/KG
Weight loss	25
Weight maintenance	30
Weight gain	35
Hypermetabolic/ malnourished	35-50

TECHNIQUE	FINDINGS

Biochemical Measurements

Obtain biochemical measures as indicated

Hemoglobin
Hematocrit
Serum albumin
Transferrin saturation
Nitrogen balance
Serum glucose
Triglycerides
Cholesterol
High-density lipoprotein
   (HDL) cholesterol
Low-density lipoprotein
   (LDL) cholesterol

EXPECTED: See reference ranges established by your particular laboratory.

AIDS TO DIFFERENTIAL DIAGNOSIS

ABNORMALITY	DESCRIPTION
Obesity	Exogenous obesity characterized by increase in number of fat cells, with excess fat located in breast, buttocks, and thighs. Associated with excessive caloric intake, thick skin, pale striae, preservation of muscle strength, and no evidence of osteoporosis. Endogenous obesity characterized by enlarged fat cells, with excess fat tissue distributed to certain regions of the body such as the trunk or abdominal areas.
Anorexia nervosa	Psychologic disorder in which the person has perceptual distortion of body shape with relentless drive for thinness through self-imposed starvation, bizarre food habits, obsessive exercise, and self-induced vomiting or laxative abuse. Adolescent and young adult women most commonly affected. Condition

Comparison of Laboratory Test Results for Anemias

TEST	NORMAL VALUE	IRON DEFICIENCY ANEMIA	FOLIC ACID DEFICIENCY ANEMIA	VITAMIN B$_{12}$ DEFICIENCY ANEMIA
Hemoglobin, 100 g/ml	Men: 14-16 Women: 12-14	Decreased	Decreased	Decreased
Hematocrit, %	Men: 40-54 Women: 37-47	Decreased	Decreased	Decreased
Mean corpuscular volume (MCV), cu μg	82-92	Decreased (<80)	Increased (>92)	Increased (>92)
Mean corpuscular hemoglobin (MCH), ρg	27-31	Decreased (<27)	Increased (>35)	Increased (>35)
Mean corpuscular hemoglobin concentration (MCHC), %	32-36	Decreased (<32)	Normal	Normal
Serum iron, μg/100 ml	60-180	Decreased	Increased	Increased
Total iron-binding capacity (TIBC), μg/100 ml	250-450	Increased (>350)	Normal	Normal
Transferrin saturation, %	20-55	Decreased (<20)	Normal	Normal

TECHNIQUE	FINDINGS
	characterized by a weight loss to 85% or less of expected weight or failure to attain expected weight. Common signs and symptoms include those of starvation.
Bulimia	Eating disorder characterized by binge eating—the rapid intake of large amount of food. Termed bulimorexia when followed by self-induced vomiting. Patient usually in late teens or early 20s; usually does not become malnourished unless body weight continues to drop to less than 85% of expected weight.
Anemias	Several types exist, depending on which nutrient is deficient; all associated with lowering of serum hemoglobin and hematocrit levels and change in size, appearance, and production of red blood cells; common symptoms include pallor, weakness, fatigue, headache, and dizziness. See table on p. 26.
Hyperlipidemia	High blood cholesterol defined as value above which risk for coronary heart disease rises. See box below and on p. 28.

Risk Factors for Coronary Heart Disease

POSITIVE

- Age: Male ≥45 years
      Female: ≥55 years or premature menopause without estrogen replacement therapy
- Family history of premature coronary heart disease
- Smoking
- Hypertension
- HDL cholesterol <35 mg/100 ml
- Diabetes

NEGATIVE

- HDL cholesterol ≥60

Data from National Institutes of Health, September 1993.

Diagnosis of Hyperlipidemia Based on LDL Cholesterol Level and Risk Factors Present

	LDL LEVEL
Without coronary heart disease (CHD) and with fewer than two risk factors	>160 mg/100 ml
Without CHD and with two or more risk factors	>130 mg/100 ml
With CHD	>100 mg/100 ml

Data from National Institutes of Health, September 1993.

PEDIATRIC VARIATIONS
EXAMINATION

TECHNIQUE	FINDINGS
Measure head circumference	
Wrap the measuring tape snugly around the infant's head at the occipital protuberance and supraorbital prominence.	Refer to growth charts for infants and children.

Pediatric patients: 1000 kcal + 100 kcal per year of age, up to age 12

Fat: Over age 2 years: less than 30% of daily calories from fat; before age 2: fat intake of 35% to 40% of calories

Protein: 0.8 g per kilogram of body weight

SAMPLE DOCUMENTATION

Male, age 45. Height: 173 cm (68 inches). Weight: 90.9 k (220 lb), 123% of desirable body weight. BMI: 30.5; triceps skinfold thickness: 20 mm, 90th percentile; mid upper arm circumference: 327.8 mm; midarm muscle circumference: 265 mm, 25th percentile; 2200 calories estimated for appropriate weight loss; 72 g protein estimated for daily needs.

CHAPTER 4

SKIN, HAIR, AND NAILS

EQUIPMENT

- Centimeter ruler (flexible, clear)
- Wood's lamp
- Flashlight with transilluminator
- Magnifying glass (optional)

EXAMINATION

TECHNIQUE	FINDINGS

Skin

Perform overall inspection of entire body

In particular, check areas not usually exposed and intertriginous surfaces.

EXPECTED: Skin color differences among body areas and between sun-exposed and non–sun-exposed areas.
UNEXPECTED: Lesions.

Inspect skin of each body area and mucous membranes

- *Color/uniformity*
  Inspect sclerae, conjunctivae, buccal mucosa, tongue, lips, nail beds, and palms of dark-skinned patients for color hues.

EXPECTED: General uniformity: dark brown to light tan, with pink or yellow overtones. Sun-darkened areas. Darker skin around knees and elbows. Callused areas yellow. Knuckles darker and palms/soles lighter in dark-skinned patients. Vascular-flush areas pink or red, especially with anxiety or excitement. Pigmented nevi. Nonpigmented striae. Freckles. Birthmarks.

Purpura—red-purple nonblanchable discoloration greater than 0.5 cm diameter.
Cause: Intravascular defects, infection

Petechiae—red-purple nonblanchable discoloration less than 0.5 cm diameter
Cause: Intravascular defects, infection

Ecchymoses—red-purple nonblanchable discoloration of variable size
Cause: Vascular wall destruction, trauma, vasculitis

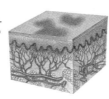

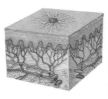

Spider angioma—red central body with radiating spiderlike legs that blanch with pressure to the central body
Cause: Liver disease, vitamin B deficiency, idiopathic

Venous star—bluish spider, linear or irregularly shaped; does not blanch with pressure
Cause: Increased pressure in superficial veins

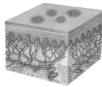

Telangiectasia—fine, irregular red line
Cause: Dilation of capillaries

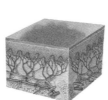

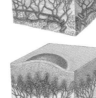

Capillary hemangioma (nevus flammeus)—red irregular macular patches
Cause: Dilation of dermal capillaries

TECHNIQUE	**FINDINGS**
	UNEXPECTED: Dysplastic, precancerous, or cancerous nevi. Chloasma. Unpigmented skin. Generalized or localized color changes. Vascular skin lesions. Vascular changes.
■ *Thickness*	**EXPECTED:** Thickness variations, with eyelids thinnest, areas of rubbing thickest. Calluses on hands and feet.

Cutaneous Color Changes			
COLOR	**CAUSE**	**DISTRIBUTION**	**SELECT CONDITIONS**
Brown	Darkening of melanin pigment	Generalized	Pituitary, adrenal, liver disease
		Localized	Nevi, neurofibromatosis
White	Absence of melanin	Generalized	Albinism
		Localized	Vitiligo
Red (erythema)	Increased cutaneous blood flow	Localized	Inflammation
		Generalized	Fever, viral exanthems, urticaria
	Increased intravascular red blood cells	Generalized	Polycythemia
Yellow	Increased bile pigmentation (jaundice)	Generalized	Liver disease
	Increased carotene pigmentation	Generalized (except sclera)	Hypothyroidism, increased intake of vegetables containing carotene
	Decreased visibility of oxyhemoglobin	Generalized	Anemia, chronic renal disease
Blue	Increased unsaturated hemoglobin secondary to hypoxia	Lips, mouth, nail beds	Cardiovascular and pulmonary diseases

TECHNIQUE	FINDINGS
	UNEXPECTED: Atrophy. Hyperkeratosis.
■ *Symmetry*	**EXPECTED:** Bilateral symmetry.

TECHNIQUE	FINDINGS

■ *Hygiene*

EXPECTED: Clean.

Palpate skin

■ *Moisture*

EXPECTED: Minimal perspiration or oiliness. Increased perspiration (associated with activity, environment, obesity, anxiety, and excitement) noticeable on palms, scalp, forehead, and axillae.
UNEXPECTED: Damp intertriginous areas.

■ *Temperature*
Palpate with dorsal surface of hand or fingers.

EXPECTED: Cool to warm. Bilateral symmetry.

■ *Texture*

EXPECTED: Smooth, soft, and even. Roughness resulting from heavy clothing, cold weather, or soap.
UNEXPECTED: Extensive or widespread roughness.

■ *Turgor and mobility*
Gently pinch skin on forearm or in sternal area and release

EXPECTED: Resilience.
UNEXPECTED: Failure of skin to return to place quickly.

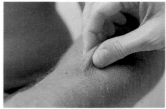

TECHNIQUE	**FINDINGS**

Inspect and palpate lesions

- *Size*
  Measure all dimensions.
- *Shape*
- *Color*
  Use Wood's lamp to distinguish fluorescing lesions.
- *Blanching*
- *Texture*
  Transilluminate to determine presence of fluid.
- *Elevation/depression*
- *Pedunculation*
- *Exudate*
  Note color, odor, amount, and consistency of lesion.
- *Configuration*
  Check lesion for annular, grouped, linear, arciform, or diffuse arrangement.
- *Location/distribution*
  Check lesion for generalized/localized, body region, patterns, or discrete/confluent.

UNEXPECTED: See table on pp. 34-39.

Hair

Inspect hair over entire body

- *Color*

EXPECTED: Light blond to black and gray, with alterations caused by rinses, dyes, and permanents.

Text continued on p. 40

Primary Skin Lesions

DESCRIPTION	EXAMPLES

MACULE

A flat, circumscribed area that is a change in the color of the skin; less than 1 cm in diameter

Freckles, flat moles (nevi), petechiae, measles, scarlet fever

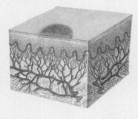

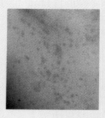

Measles. *(From Habif, 1996.)*

PAPULE

An elevated, firm, circumscribed area less than 1 cm in diameter

Wart (verruca), elevated moles, lichen planus

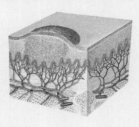

Lichen planus. *(From Weston, Lane, Morelli, 1996.)*

Primary Skin Lesions—cont'd

DESCRIPTION	EXAMPLES

PATCH

A flat, nonpalpable, irregular-shaped macule more than 1 cm in diameter

Vitiligo, port-wine stains, mongolian spots, café au lait spots

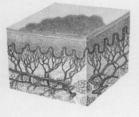

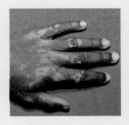

Vitiligo. *(From Weston, Lane, and Morelli, 1991.)*

PLAQUE

Elevated, firm, and rough lesion with flat top surface greater than 1 cm in diameter

Psoriasis, seborrheic and actinic keratoses

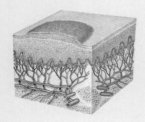

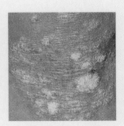

Plaque. *(From Habif, 1996.)*

Continued

Primary Skin Lesions—cont'd	
DESCRIPTION	**EXAMPLES**

WHEAL

Elevated irregular-shaped area of cutaneous edema; solid, transient; variable diameter

Insect bites, urticaria, allergic reaction

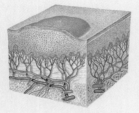

Wheal. *(From Farrar et al, 1992.)*

NODULE

Elevated, firm, circumscribed lesion; deeper in dermis than a papule; 1 to 2 cm in diameter

Erythema nodosum, lipomas

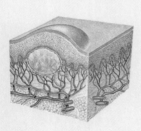

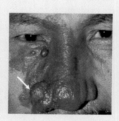

Hypertrophic nodule. *(From Goldman and Fitzpatrick, 1994.)*

Primary Skin Lesions—cont'd

DESCRIPTION	EXAMPLES

TUMOR

Elevated and solid lesion; may or may not be clearly demarcated; deeper in dermis; greater than 2 cm in diameter

Neoplasms, benign tumor, lipoma, hemangioma

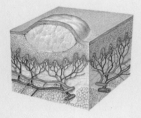

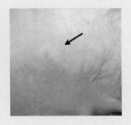

Hemangioma. *(From Weston, Lane, Morelli, 1996.)*

VESICLE

Elevated, circumscribed, superficial, not into dermis; filled with serous fluid; less than 1 cm in diameter

Varicella (chicken pox), herpes zoster (shingles)

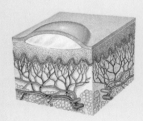

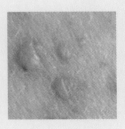

Vesicles caused by varicella. *(From Farrar et al, 1992.)*

Continued

Primary Skin Lesions—cont'd

DESCRIPTION	EXAMPLES

BULLA

Vesicle greater than 1 cm in diameter

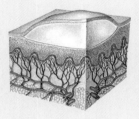

Blister, pemphigus vulgaris

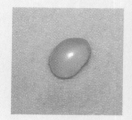

Blister. *(From White, 1994.)*

PUSTULE

Elevated, superficial lesion; similar to a vesicle but filled with purulent fluid

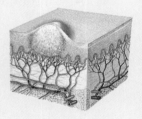

Impetigo, acne

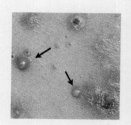

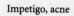
Acne. *(From Weston, Lane, Morelli, 1996.)*

Primary Skin Lesions—cont'd

DESCRIPTION	EXAMPLES

CYST

Elevated, circumscribed, encapsulated lesion; in dermis or subcutaneous layer; filled with liquid or semisolid material

Sebaceous cyst, cystic acne

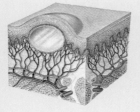

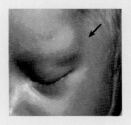

Sebaceous cyst. *(From Weston, Lane, Morelli, 1996.)*

TELANGIECTASIA

Fine, irregular red lines produced by capillary dilation

Telangiectasia in rosacea

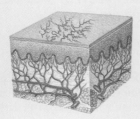

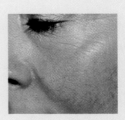

Telangiectasia. *(From Goldman and Fitzpatrick, 1994.)*

TECHNIQUE	FINDINGS

■ *Distribution/quantity*

EXPECTED: Hair present on scalp, lower face, neck, nares, ears, chest, axillae, back and shoulders, arms, legs, pubic areas, and around nipples. Scalp hair loss in adult men, adrenal androgenic female-pattern alopecia in adult women.

UNEXPECTED: Localized or generalized hair loss, inflammation or scarring. Broken/absent hair shafts. Hirsutism in women.

Palpate for texture

EXPECTED: Coarse or fine, curly or straight, shiny, smooth, and resilient. Fine vellus covering body; coarse terminal hair on scalp, pubic, and axillary areas and in male beard.

UNEXPECTED: Dryness and brittleness.

Nails

Inspect nails

■ *Color*

EXPECTED: Variations of pink with varying opacity. Pigment deposits in persons with dark skin. White spots.

UNEXPECTED: Yellow or green-black discoloration. Diffuse darkening. Pigment deposits in persons with light skin. Longitudinal red, brown, or white streaks, or white bands. White, yellow, or green tinge.

TECHNIQUE	FINDINGS

■ *Length/configuration/symmetry*

EXPECTED: Varying shape, smooth and flat/slightly convex, with edges smooth and rounded.
UNEXPECTED: Jagged, broken, or bitten edges or cuticles. Peeling. Absence of nail.

■ *Cleanliness*

EXPECTED: Clean and neat.
UNEXPECTED: Unkempt.

■ *Ridging and beading*

EXPECTED: Longitudinal ridging and beading.
UNEXPECTED: Longitudinal ridging and grooving with lichen planus. Transverse grooving, rippling, and depressions. Pitting.

Palpate nail plate

■ *Texture/firmness/thickness/uniformity*

EXPECTED: Hard and smooth with uniform thickness.
UNEXPECTED: Thickening or thinning.

■ *Adherence to nail bed*
Gently squeeze between thumb and finger.

EXPECTED: Firmness.
UNEXPECTED: Separation. Boggy nail base.

Measure nail base angle

Inspect fingers when patient places dorsal surfaces of fingertips together.

EXPECTED: 160-degree angle.
UNEXPECTED: Clubbing.

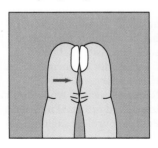

Expected finding

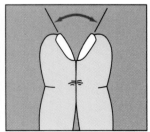

Clubbing

TECHNIQUE	FINDINGS

Inspect and palpate proximal and lateral nail fold

UNEXPECTED: Redness, swelling, pus, warts, cysts, tumors, and pain.

AIDS TO DIFFERENTIAL DIAGNOSIS

ABNORMALITY	DESCRIPTION
Corn (clavus)	Flat or slightly elevated, circumscribed, painful lesions. Smooth, hard surface. Soft corns: whitish thickenings. Hard corns: sharply delineated, conical.
Callus	Superficial area of hyperkeratosis. Less demarcated than corns. Usually nontender.
Tinea (dermatophytosis)	Papular, pustular, vesicular, erythematous, or scaling lesions. Possible secondary bacterial infection.
Basal cell carcinoma	Cutaneous neoplasm in nodular, pigmented, cystic, sclerosing, superficial, and other forms.
Kaposi sarcoma	Soft, vascular, bluish purple, painless lesions. Macular or papular. May appear as plaques, keloids, or ecchymotic areas.
Eczematous dermatitis	Acute: erythematous, pruritic, weeping vesicles, often excoriated and crusted from scratching. Subacute: erythema and scaling, possible itching. Chronic: thick, lichenified, pruritic plaques.
Paronychia	Redness, swelling, tenderness at lateral and proximal nail folds. Possible purulent drainage under cuticle. Acute or chronic (with nail rippling).

ABNORMALITY	DESCRIPTION
Ingrown nail	Pain and swelling resulting from nail piercing fold and growing into dermis.

PEDIATRIC VARIATIONS

EXAMINATION

TECHNIQUE	FINDINGS

Skin

Inspect the hands and feet of newborns for skin creases

	EXPECTED: Number of creases is indication of maturity of the newborn; the greater the gestational age, the more creases.
	UNEXPECTED: A single transverse crease across the palm frequently seen in infants with Down syndrome.

AIDS TO DIFFERENTIAL DIAGNOSIS

ABNORMALITY	DESCRIPTION
Café au lait spots	Coffee-colored multiple patches, diameter more than 1 cm.
Seborrheic dermatitis	Thick, yellow, adherent crusted scalp, ear, or neck lesions.
Impetigo	Honey-colored crusted or ruptured vesicles.
Miliaria ("prickly heat")	Irregular, red, macular rash.
Reddened patches	Irregular reddened areas suggestive of richer capillary bed. Include strawberry hemangioma and cavernous hemangioma.
Chicken pox (varicella)	Fever, mild malaise, and pruritic maculopapular skin eruption that becomes vesicular in a matter of hours.

ABNORMALITY	DESCRIPTION
German measles (rubella)	Generalized light pink to red maculopapular rash, low-grade fever, coryza, sore throat, cough.

SAMPLE DOCUMENTATION

Skin. Dark brown, smooth with a 2 cm white scar at the inferior aspect of R scapula; no keloids. Turgor resilient, skin uniform and dry. No edema evident. Multiple 2 to 4 mm round vesicles, discrete and confluent in a linear pattern over the dorsal aspect of L ankle and lower leg; 3 to 4 mm surrrounding erythema. No exudate, swelling, or temperature changes.

Hair. Curly, black, thick with female distribution pattern. Texture coarse.

Nails. Opaque, short, and well groomed; uniform and without deformities. Nail beds pink. Nail base angle 160 degrees. No redness, exudate, or swelling in the surrounding folds, and no tenderness to palpation.

CHAPTER 5

LYMPHATIC SYSTEM

EQUIPMENT
- Centimeter ruler
- Skin-marking pencil

EXAMINATION

The lymphatic system is examined by inspection and palpation, region by region, during the examination of other body systems, as well as with palpation of the spleen.

The Lymph Nodes Most Accessible to Inspection and Palpation

Obviously, the more superficial the node, the more accessible.

THE "NECKLACE" OF NODES

Parotid and retropharyngeal
  (tonsillar)
Submandibular
Submental
Sublingual (facial)
Superficial anterior cervical
Superficial posterior cervical
Preauricular and postauricular
Occipital
Supraclavicular

THE ARMS

Axillary
Epitrochlear (cubital)

THE LEGS

Superficial superior inguinal
Superficial inferior inguinal
Occasionally, popliteal

TECHNIQUE	FINDINGS

Head and Neck

Inspect visible nodes

Ask if patient is aware of any lumps.

UNEXPECTED: Edema, erythema, red streaks, or lesions.

TECHNIQUE   **FINDINGS**

Palpate for superficial nodes; note size, consistency, mobility, tenderness, warmth

Bend patient's head
slightly forward or to the
side. Palpate gently with
pads of second, third, and
fourth fingers.

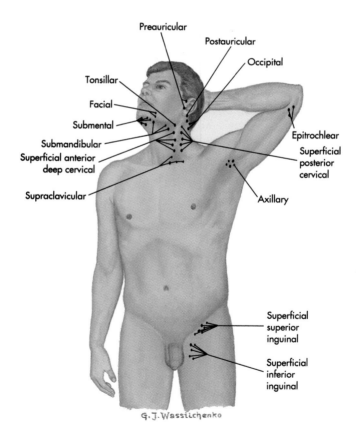

G.J.Wassilchenko

TECHNIQUE   **FINDINGS**

Head/Neck

- *Occipital nodes at base of skull*
- *Postauricular nodes over mastoid process*
- *Preauricular nodes in front of ears*
- *Parotid and retropharyngeal nodes at angle of mandible*
- *Submandibular nodes between angle and tip of mandible*
- *Submental nodes behind tip of mandible*

EXPECTED: Nodes accessible to palpation but not large or firm enough to be felt.
UNEXPECTED: Enlarged, tender, red or discolored, fixed, matted, inflamed, or warm nodes, and increased vascularity.

Neck

- *Superficial cervical nodes at sternocleidomastoid*

EXPECTED: Nodes accessible to palpation but not large or firm enough to be felt.

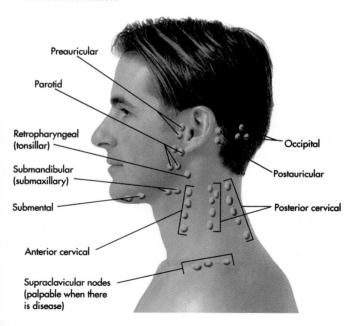

Preauricular

Parotid

Retropharyngeal (tonsillar)

Submandibular (submaxillary)

Submental

Anterior cervical

Supraclavicular nodes (palpable when there is disease)

Occipital

Postauricular

Posterior cervical

TECHNIQUE	FINDINGS

- *Posterior cervical nodes along anterior border of trapezius*
- *Deep cervical nodes along anterior border of trapezius*
- *Supraclavicular areas*
  If enlarged nodes are found, inspect regions drained by the nodes for infection or malignancy and examine other regions for enlargement.

UNEXPECTED: Enlarged, tender, red or discolored, fixed, matted, inflamed, or warm nodes, and increased vascularity

UNEXPECTED: Detection of Virchow nodes.

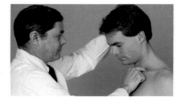

Axillae

Inspect visible nodes

Ask if patient is aware of any lumps.

UNEXPECTED: Edema, erythema, red streaks, or lesions.

Palpate superficial nodes for size, consistency, mobility, tenderness, warmth

Using firm, deliberate, gentle touch, rotate fingertips and palm. Attempt to glide fingers beneath nodes.

Axillary nodes

Support patient's forearm with your contralateral arm and bring palm of examining hand flat into axilla.

If enlarged nodes are found, inspect regions drained by the nodes for infection or malignancy and examine other regions for enlargement.

EXPECTED: Nodes accessible to palpation, but not large or firm enough to be felt.

UNEXPECTED: Enlarged, tender; red or discolored; fixed, matted; inflamed, warm; increased vascularity.

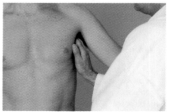

TECHNIQUE	FINDINGS

Other Lymph Nodes

Inspect visible nodes

Ask if patient is aware of any lumps.

UNEXPECTED: Edema, erythema, red streaks, or lesions.

Palpate superficial nodes for size, consistency, mobility, tenderness, warmth

Systematically palpate other areas, moving hand in circular fashion, probing without pressing hard.

■ *Epitrochlear nodes*
Support elbow in one hand while exploring with the other.

EXPECTED: Nodes accessible to palpation, but not large or firm enough to be felt.

UNEXPECTED: Enlarged, tender; red or discolored; fixed, matted; inflamed, warm; increased vascularity.

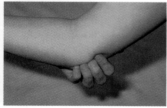

■ *Inguinal and popliteal area*
Have patient lie supine with knee slightly flexed.

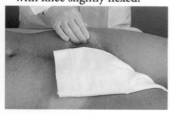

If enlarged nodes are found, inspect regions drained by the nodes for infection or malignancy and examine other regions for enlargement.

AIDS TO DIFFERENTIAL DIAGNOSIS

ABNORMALITY	DESCRIPTION
Acute lymphangitis	Pain, malaise, illness, and possibly fever. Red streak (tracing of fine lines) may follow course of lymphatic collecting duct. Inflamed area sometimes slightly indurated and palpable to gentle touch. Related infection possible distally, particularly interdigitally.
Non-Hodgkin lymphoma	Well-defined, solid neoplasm, often in lymph nodes or spleen.
Hodgkin disease	Painless, inexorably progressive enlargement of cervical lymph nodes. Generally asymmetric. Nodes sometimes matted and generally very firm, almost rubbery. Nodes sometimes produce pressure on surrounding structures, prompting need for medical care.

Some Conditions Simulating Lymph Node Enlargement

Lymphangioma
Hemangioma (tends to feel spongy; appears reddish blue, depending on size and extent of angiomatous involvement)
Branchial cleft cyst (sometimes accompanied by a tiny orifice in the neck on a line extending to the ear)
Thyroglossal duct cyst
Laryngocele
Esophageal diverticulum
Thyroid goiter
Graves disease
Hashimoto thyroiditis
Parotid swelling (e.g., from mumps or tumor)

ABNORMALITY	DESCRIPTION
Epstein-Barr virus; mononucleosis	Pharyngitis, fever, fatigue, and malaise. Frequently splenomegaly and/or rash. Palpable nodes generalized, but more commonly in anterior and posterior cervical chains. Nodes vary in firmness, are generally discrete, and are occasionally tender.
Streptococcal pharyngitis	Sore throat. Often runny nose. Sometimes headache, fatigue, and abdominal pain. Firm, discrete, often tender anterior cervical nodes generally felt.
Herpes simplex	Often discrete labial and gingival ulcers, high fever, and enlargement of anterior cervical and submandibular nodes. Nodes tend to be firm, quite discrete, movable, and tender.
Acquired immune deficiency syndrome (AIDS)	Recurrent, often severe, opportunistic infections. Initially: lymphadenopathy, fatigue, fever, and weight loss.
Human immunodeficiency virus (HIV) seropositivity	Warning signs include severe fatigue, malaise, weakness, persistent unexplained weight loss, persistent lymphadenopathy, fevers, arthralgias, and persistent diarrhea.

PEDIATRIC VARIATIONS

EXAMINATION

TECHNIQUE	FINDINGS
Head and Neck	
Palpate for superficial nodes	
■ *Occipital nodes at base of skull* ■ *Postauricular nodes over mastoid process*	**EXPECTED:** In children, small, firm, discrete, nontender, nonmovable nodes in occipital, postauricular chains.

TECHNIQUE	FINDINGS

Other Lymph Nodes

Palpate superficial nodes

■ *Inguinal and popliteal area* **EXPECTED:** In children, small, firm, discrete nodes; nontender, movable in inguinal chain.

SAMPLE DOCUMENTATION

No visible enlargement of lymph nodes in any area. On palpation, enlarged node (2 cm in diameter) in left posterior cervical triangle, firm, nontender, movable, no overlying warmth, erythema, or edema. In addition, a few shotty nodes palpated in posterior cervical triangles bilaterally and in femoral chains bilaterally.

CHAPTER 6

HEAD AND NECK

EQUIPMENT

- Tape measure
- Stethoscope
- Cup of water
- Transilluminator

EXAMINATION

Ask patient to sit.

TECHNIQUE

FINDINGS

Head and Face

Observe head position

EXPECTED: Upright, midline, and still.

UNEXPECTED: Horizontal jerking or bobbing, nodding, tilted.

Inspect facial features

- *Shape*
  Observe eyelids; eyebrows; palpebral fissures; nasolabial folds; and mouth at rest, during movement, and with expression.

EXPECTED: Variations according to race, sex, and body build.

UNEXPECTED: Change in shape. Unusual features: edema, puffiness, coarsened features, prominent eyes, hirsutism, lack of expression, excessive perspiration, pallor, or pigmentation variations. Tics.

TECHNIQUE	FINDINGS

■ *Symmetry*
Note if asymmetry affects all features of one side or a portion of face.

EXPECTED: Slight asymmetry.
UNEXPECTED: Facial nerve paralysis, facial nerve weakness, or problem with peripheral trigeminal nerve.

■ *Characteristic facies*

Inspect skull and scalp

■ *Size/shape/symmetry*

EXPECTED: Symmetric.

■ *Scalp condition*
Systematically part hair from frontal to occipital region.

UNEXPECTED: Lesions, scabs, tenderness, parasites, nits, scaliness.

■ *Hair pattern*
Pay special attention to areas behind ears, at hairline, and at crown.

EXPECTED: Bitemporal recession or balding over crown in men.

Palpate head and scalp

■ *Symmetry*
Palpate in gentle, rotary motion from front to back.

EXPECTED: Symmetric and smooth with bones indistinguishable. Ridge of sagittal occasionally palpable.
UNEXPECTED: Indentations or depressions.

Palpate hair

■ *Texture/color distribution*

EXPECTED: Smooth, symmetrically distributed.
UNEXPECTED: Splitting, or cracked ends. Coarse, dry, or brittle. Fine and silky.

Palpate temporal arteries

Note course of arteries

UNEXPECTED: Thickening, hardness, or tenderness.

TECHNIQUE	FINDINGS

Auscultate temporal arteries and over skull and eyes

EXPECTED: No bruits.

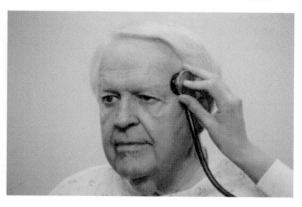

Inspect salivary glands

■ *Symmetry/size*
Palpate if asymmetry noted. Have patient open mouth and press on the salivary duct to attempt to express material.

UNEXPECTED: Asymmetry or enlargement. Tenderness. Discrete nodule.

Neck

Inspect neck

■ *Symmetry*
Inspect in usual position, in slight hyperextension, and during swallowing. Look for landmarks of anterior and posterior triangles.

EXPECTED: Bilateral symmetry of sternocleidomastoid and trapezius muscles.
UNEXPECTED: Asymmetry, torticollis.

TECHNIQUE	FINDINGS

- *Trachea*
  Inspect in usual position, in slight hyperextension, and while patient swallows.

  EXPECTED: Midline placement.

- *Condition of neck*

  UNEXPECTED: Masses, webbing, excessive posterior skinfolds, unusually short neck, distention of jugular vein, prominence of carotid arteries, or edema.

Evaluate range of motion

  Have patient flex, extend, rotate, and laterally turn head and neck.

  EXPECTED: Smooth.
  UNEXPECTED: Pain, dizziness, or limitation of motion.

Palpate neck

- *Trachea*
  Place a thumb on each side of trachea in lower portion of neck, and compare space between trachea and sternocleidomastoid on each side.

  EXPECTED: Midline position.
  UNEXPECTED: Deviation to right or left.

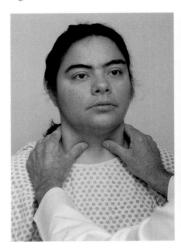

TECHNIQUE	FINDINGS

- *Hyoid bone/thyroid and cricoid cartilages*
  Have patient swallow.

  EXPECTED: Smooth. Moves during swallowing.
  UNEXPECTED: Tender.

- *Cartilaginous rings of trachea*
  Have patient swallow.

  EXPECTED: Distinct.
  UNEXPECTED: Tender.

- *Tracheal tug*
  With neck extended, palpate for movement with index finger and thumb on each side of trachea below thyroid isthmus.

  UNEXPECTED: Downward tug synchronous with pulse.

Palpate lymph nodes

- *Size/consistency, mobility/condition*

  UNEXPECTED: Enlarged, matted, tender, fixed, warm.

Palpate thyroid gland

- *Symmetry*
  Observe while patient hyperextends neck. Then observe while patient sips water while neck is hyperextended.

  UNEXPECTED: Asymmetry. Enlarged and visible thyroid gland.

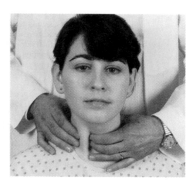

TECHNIQUE	FINDINGS

■ *Size/shape/configuration/ consistency*

Stand either facing or behind patient. Have patient hold head slightly forward and tipped toward side being examined. Lightly palpate isthmus, main body, and lateral lobes. Give water to patient to facilitate swallowing.

EXPECTED: Lobes (if felt) small and smooth. Gland rises freely with swallowing. Right lobe as much as 25% larger than left. Tissue firm and pliable.

UNEXPECTED: Enlarged, tenderness, nodules (smooth or irregular, soft or hard), coarse tissue, and gritty sensation.

If gland is enlarged, auscultate for vascular sounds with stethoscope bell.

UNEXPECTED: Bruit.

AIDS TO DIFFERENTIAL DIAGNOSIS

ABNORMALITY	DESCRIPTION
Myxedema	Dull, puffy, yellow skin. Coarse, sparse hair. Temporal loss of eyebrows. Periorbital edema. Prominent tongue. Hypothyroidism (see p. 59).
Graves disease	Diffuse thyroid enlargement, hyperthyroidism. Various pathologic conditions: ophthalmologic (prominent eyes, lid retraction, staring or startled expression), dermatologic (fine and moist skin, fine hair), and musculoskeletal (muscle weakness).
Down syndrome	Depressed nasal bridge, epicanthal folds, mongoloid slant of eyes, low-set ears, large tongue.

Hyperthyroidism Versus Hypothyroidism

SYSTEM OR STRUCTURE AFFECTED	HYPERTHYROIDISM	HYPOTHYROIDISM
Constitutional		
Temperature preference	Cool climate	Warm climate
Weight	Loss	Gain
Emotional state	Nervous, easily irritated, highly energetic	Lethargic, complacent, disinterested
Hair	Fine, with hair loss; failure to hold a permanent wave	Coarse, with tendency to break
Skin	Warm, fine, hyperpigmentation at pressure points	Coarse, scaling, dry
Fingernails	Thin, with tendency to break; may show onycholysis	Thick
Eyes	Bilateral or unilateral proptosis, lid retraction, double vision	Puffiness in periorbital region
Neck	Goiter, change in shirt neck size, pain over thyroid	No goiter
Cardiac	Tachycardia, arrhythmia, palpitations	No change noted
Gastrointestinal	Increased frequency of bowel movements; diarrhea rare	Constipation
Menstrual	Scant flow, amenorrhea	Menorrhagia
Neuromuscular	Increasing weakness, especially of proximal muscles	Lethargic, but good muscular strength

Headaches

Headaches are one of the most common complaints and probably one of the most self-medicated. They are not always benign. A history of insistent headache, severe and recurrent, must always be given attention. Sometimes the underlying cause is life threatening, such as a brain tumor. Sometimes it is life intimidating, such as migraines. At other times it is easily confronted, such as when it is the result of drinking wine. The patient's history is fully as important as the physical examination in getting at the root of a headache. Various kinds of headaches can be compared as follows.

CHARACTERISTIC	CLASSIC MIGRAINE	COMMON MIGRAINE	CLUSTER	HYPERTENSIVE	MUSCULAR, TENSION	TEMPORAL ARTERITIS
Age at onset	Childhood	Childhood	Adulthood	Adulthood	Adulthood	Older adulthood
Location	Unilateral	Generalized	Unilateral	Bilateral or occipital	Unilateral or bilateral	Unilateral or bilateral
Duration	Hour to days	Hours to days	$1/2$ to 2 hours	Hours	Hours to days	Hours to days
Time of onset	Morning or night	Morning or night	Night	Morning	Anytime, commonly in afternoon or evening	Anytime
Quality of pain	Pulsating or throbbing	Pulsating or throbbing	Intense burning, boring, searing, knifelike	Throbbing	Bandlike, constricting	Throbbing

Prodromal event	Well-defined neurologic event, scotoma, aphasia, hemianopsia, aura	Vague neurologic changes, personality change, fluid retention, appetite loss	Personality changes, sleep disturbances	None	None	None
Precipitating event	Menstrual period, missing meals, birth control pills, letdown after stress	Menstrual period, missing meals, birth control pills, letdown after stress	Alcohol consumption	None	Stress, anger, bruxism	None
Frequency	Twice a week	Twice a week	Several times nightly for several nights, then none	Daily	Daily	Daily
Gender predilection	Females	Females	Males	Equal	Equal	Equal
Other symptoms	Nausea, vomiting	Nausea, vomiting	Increased lacrimation, nasal discharge	Generally remits as day progresses	None	None

EXAMINATION

TECHNIQUE	FINDINGS

Head and Face

Palpate head and scalp

- *Symmetry* — **EXPECTED:** An infant's head circumference is 2 cm greater than chest circumference up to the age of 2 years.

  In infants, transilluminate the skull — **EXPECTED:** 2 cm ring of light.

- *Skull condition* — **EXPECTED:** In infants, posterior fontanels closed at birth; anterior fontanels closed at 18 to 24 months.

  UNEXPECTED: Tenderness or depressions, sunken areas; swelling, bulging, or depressed fontanels.

- *Scalp* — **EXPECTED:** Free movement.

  UNEXPECTED: Fixation of scalp, bulging either on one side or crossing the midline of the scalp.

Percuss the skull

EXPECTED: Macewen sign, cracked-pot sound, is physiologic when fontanels are open.

UNEXPECTED: Macewen sign may indicate increased intracranial pressure after fontanel closure.

TECHNIQUE	FINDINGS

Auscultate temporal arteries and over skull and eyes

EXPECTED: Bruits are common in children up to age 5 years.

Neck

Palpate thyroid gland

■ *Symmetry*

EXPECTED: In children, thyroid gland may be palpable.

SAMPLE DOCUMENTATION

Head. Held erect and midline. Skull normocephalic, symmetric, and smooth without deformities. Facial features symmetric. No frontal or maxillary sinus tenderness elicited with palpation or percussion. Salivary glands not inflamed or tender. Temporal artery pulsations visible bilaterally, soft and nontender to palpation. No bruits.

Neck. Trachea midline. No jugular venous distention (JVD) or carotid artery prominence. Thyroid palpable, firm, smooth, not enlarged. Thyroid and cartilages move with swallowing. No nodules or tenderness. No bruits. Full range of motion (ROM) of the neck without discomfort.

CLINICAL AND
REFERENCE NOTES

CHAPTER 7

EYES

EQUIPMENT

- Snellen chart or E chart
- Eye cover, gauze, or opaque card
- Rosenbaum or Jaeger near-vision card
- Penlight
- Cotton wisp
- Ophthalmoscope

EXAMINATION

Ask patient to sit or stand.

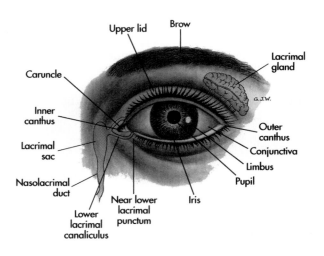

TECHNIQUE	FINDINGS

Visual Testing

Measure visual acuity

- *Distance vision*
  Use Snellen test or **E** chart. If tested with and without corrective lenses, test without lenses first and record readings separately.

EXPECTED: Vision 20/20 with or without lenses with near and far vision in each eye.
UNEXPECTED: Myopia, amblyopia, or presbyopia.

- *Near vision*
  Use near-vision card.
- *Peripheral vision*
  Test nasal, temporal, superior, and inferior fields by moving your finger into field from outside.

UNEXPECTED: Fields of vision more limited than 60 degrees nasally, 90 degrees temporally, 50 degrees superiorly, and 70 degrees inferiorly.

External Examination

Inspect eyebrows

- *Size/extension*

EXPECTED: Unusually thin if plucked.
UNEXPECTED: End short of temporal canthus.

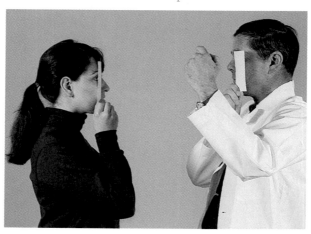

TECHNIQUE	FINDINGS
■ *Hair texture*	**UNEXPECTED:** Coarse.
Inspect orbital area	
	UNEXPECTED: Edema, puffiness not related to aging, or sagging tissue below orbit. Xanthelasma.
Inspect eyelids	
■ *Eyelid position*	**UNEXPECTED:** Ectropion or entropion.
■ *Ability to open wide and close completely* Examine with eyes lightly closed, closed completely, and open wide.	**EXPECTED:** Superior eyelid covering a portion of iris when open. **UNEXPECTED:** Fasciculations when lightly closed. Ptosis. Lagophthalmos.
■ *Eyelid margin*	**UNEXPECTED:** Flakiness, redness, or swelling. Hordeola.
■ *Eyelashes*	**EXPECTED:** Present on both lids. Turned outward.
Palpate eyelids	
	UNEXPECTED: Nodules.
Palpate the eye	
	EXPECTED: Can be gently pushed into orbit without discomfort. **UNEXPECTED:** Firm and resists palpation.

TECHNIQUE	FINDINGS

Pull down lower lids and inspect conjunctivae and sclerae

- *Color*
Inspect upper tarsal conjunctivae only if presence of foreign body is suspected.

EXPECTED: Conjunctivae clear and inapparent. Sclerae white and visible above irides only when eyelids are wide open.
UNEXPECTED: Conjunctivae with erythema. Sclerae yellow or green. Sclerae with dark, rust-colored pigment anterior to insertion of medial rectus muscle.

- *Condition*

UNEXPECTED: Exudate. Pterygium. Corneal arcus senilis or opacities.

Inspect lacrimal gland region

- *Lacrimal gland puncta*
Palpate lower orbital rim near inner canthus. If temporal aspect of upper lid feels full, evert lid and inspect gland.

EXPECTED: Slight elevations with central depression on both upper and lower lid margins.
UNEXPECTED: Enlarged glands. Dry eyes.

Test corneal sensitivity

Touch wisp of cotton to cornea.

EXPECTED: A bilateral blink reflex.

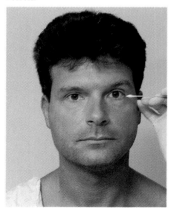

TECHNIQUE	FINDINGS

Inspect external eyes

- *Corneal clarity*
  Shine light tangentially on cornea.
  UNEXPECTED: Blood vessels present.
- *Irides*
  EXPECTED: Clearly visible pattern. Similar color.
- *Pupillary size/shape*
  EXPECTED: Round, regular, and equal in size.
  UNEXPECTED: Miosis, mydriasis, anisocoria, or coloboma.
- *Pupillary response to light*
  EXPECTED: Constricting with consensual response of opposite pupil.
- *Pupillary accommodation*
  EXPECTED: Constricting when pupils focus on near object or dilating when focus changes from near to distant.

Extraocular Eye Muscles

Evaluate muscle balance and movement of eyes

- *Six cardinal fields of gaze*
  Hold patient's chin and ask patient to watch finger or penlight.
  EXPECTED: A few horizontal nystagmic beats. Smooth, full, coordinated movement of eyes.
  UNEXPECTED: Sustained or jerking nystagmus. Exposure of sclera from lid lag.

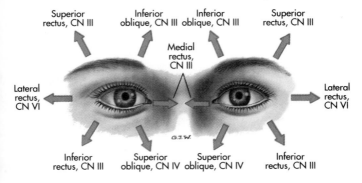

TECHNIQUE	FINDINGS

■ *Corneal light reflex*
  Direct light to nasal bridge from 30 cm (12 in). Have patient look at nearby object.

EXPECTED: Light reflected symmetrically from both eyes.

■ *Cover-uncover test*
  Perform if imbalance found with corneal light reflex test. Have patient stare ahead at near, fixed object. Cover one eye and observe other; remove cover and observe uncovered eye. Repeat with other eye.

UNEXPECTED: Movement of covered or uncovered eye.

Ophthalmoscopic Examination
Inspect internal eye

■ *Lens clarity*
■ *Anterior chamber*
  Shine focused light tangentially at limbus. Note illumination of iris nasally.

UNEXPECTED: Shallow chamber. If observed, avoid mydriatics.

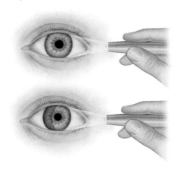

TECHNIQUE	FINDINGS

- *Use the ophthalmoscope*
  With patient looking at distant object, direct light at pupil from about 30 cm (12 in). Move toward patient, observing:
  - *Red reflex*
  - *Fundus*

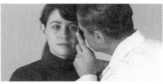

UNEXPECTED: Opacities.
EXPECTED: Yellow or pink background, depending on race. Possible crescents or dots of pigment at disc margin, usually temporally.
UNEXPECTED: Discrete areas of pigmentation away from the disc. Lesions. Drusen bodies. Hemorrhages.

- *Blood vessel characteristics*
  Follow blood vessels distally in each quadrant noting crossings of arterioles and venules.

EXPECTED: Possible venous pulsations (should be documented). Arteriole/venule (A/V) ratio 3:5 or 2:3.
UNEXPECTED: Glaucomatous cupping, nicking, crossing, tortuosity.

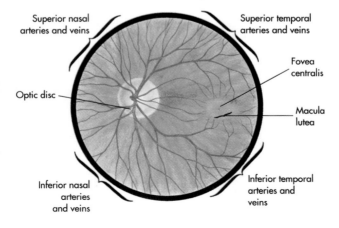

Superior nasal arteries and veins

Superior temporal arteries and veins

Fovea centralis

Optic disc

Macula lutea

Inferior nasal arteries and veins

Inferior temporal arteries and veins

TECHNIQUE	FINDINGS
■ *Disc characteristics*	**EXPECTED:** Yellow to creamy pink, varying by race. Sharp, well-defined margin, especially in temporal region. 1.5 mm diameter. **UNEXPECTED:** Myelinated nerve fibers. Papilledema. Glaucomatous cupping.
■ *Macula densa characteristics* Ask patient to look directly at light.	**EXPECTED:** Yellow dot surrounded by deep pink.

AIDS TO DIFFERENTIAL DIAGNOSIS

ABNORMALITY	DESCRIPTION
Strabismus (paralytic and nonparalytic)	Eyes do not focus simultaneously. Can focus separately in nonparalytic type.
Episcleritis	Inflammation of superficial layers of sclera anterior to insertion of rectus muscles. Generally localized with purplish elevation of a few millimeters.
Cataracts	Opacity of lens, generally central, occasionally peripheral.
Diabetic retinopathy (background)	Dot hemorrhages or microaneurysms. Hard exudates (bright yellow, sharply defined borders) and soft exudates (dull yellow spots, poorly defined margins).

PEDIATRIC VARIATIONS

EXAMINATION

TECHNIQUE	FINDINGS

Visual Testing

Measure visual acuity

■ *Distance vision*

Visual acuity is tested, when the child is cooperative, with the Snellen **E** or picture chart, usually about 3 years of age.

EXPECTED:

AGE (YEARS)	ACUITY
3	20/50
4	20/40
5	20/30
6	20/20

Infants should be able to focus on and track a face or light through 60 degrees.

Extraocular Eye Muscles

Evaluate muscle balance and movement of eyes

Evaluation of six cardinal fields of gaze is performed as with adults. You may, however, need to hold the child's head still.

SAMPLE DOCUMENTATION

Eyes. Near vision 20/40 in each eye uncorrected, corrected to 20/20 with glasses. Distant vision 20/20 by Snellen. Visual fields full by confrontation. Extraocular movements intact and full, no nystagmus. Corneal light reflex equal.

Lids and globes are symmetrical. No ptosis. Eyebrows full, no edema or lesions evident.

Conjunctivae pink, sclerae clear. No discharge evident. Cornea clear, corneal reflex intact. Irides brown, pupils equal, round, and reactive to light and accommodation.

Ophthalmoscopic examination reveals a red reflex. Discs cream colored, borders well defined with temporal pigmentation in each eye (OU). No venous pulsations evident at the disc. Arteriole/venule ratio is 3:5, no nicking or crossing changes, hemorrhages, or exudates noted. Maculae are yellow OU.

CLINICAL AND
REFERENCE NOTES

CHAPTER 8

Ears, Nose, and Throat

EQUIPMENT

- Otoscope with pneumatic attachment
- Tuning fork
- Nasal speculum
- Tongue blades
- Gloves
- Gauze
- Penlight, sinus transilluminator, or light from otoscope

EXAMINATION

Have patient sit.

TECHNIQUE	FINDINGS

Ears

Inspect auricles and mastoid area

Examine lateral and medical surfaces and surrounding tissue.

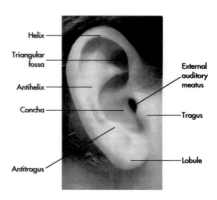

Helix

Triangular fossa

Antihelix

Concha

Antitragus

External auditory meatus

Tragus

Lobule

TECHNIQUE	FINDINGS
■ *Size/shape/symmetry*	**EXPECTED:** Familial variations. Auricles of equal size and similar appearance.
	UNEXPECTED: Unequal size or configuration. Cauliflower ear and other deformities.
■ *Landmarks*	**EXPECTED:** Darwin tubercle or preauricular pits.
	UNEXPECTED: Moles, cysts or other lesions, nodules, or tophi. Openings in preauricular area.
■ *Color*	**EXPECTED:** Same color as facial skin.
	UNEXPECTED: Blueness, pallor, or excessive redness.
■ *Position* Draw imaginary line between outer canthus and most prominent protuberance of occiput. Draw imaginary line perpendicular to first line and anterior to auricle.	**EXPECTED:** Top of auricle touching or above line.
	UNEXPECTED: Auricle positioned below line; unequal alignment.
	EXPECTED: Vertical position.
	UNEXPECTED: Lateral posterior angle greater than 10 degrees.
■ *Preauricular area*	**EXPECTED:** Skin smooth.
	UNEXPECTED: Discharge.
■ *External auditory canal*	**EXPECTED:** No discharge; canal walls pink.
	UNEXPECTED: Serous, bloody, or purulent discharge, foul smell.

Palpate auricles and mastoid area

EXPECTED: Firm and mobile, readily recoiling from folded position; nontender.

TECHNIQUE	FINDINGS
	UNEXPECTED: Tenderness, swelling, nodules. Pain from pulling on lobule.

Inspect auditory canal with otoscope

Tilt patient's head toward opposite shoulder. Pull auricle upward and back while *gently* inserting speculum. Assess canal from meatus to tympanic membrane.	**EXPECTED:** Cerumen in varying color and texture. Pink canal. Hairs in the outer third of the canal. **UNEXPECTED:** Cerumen obscures tympanic membrane, odor, lesions, discharge, scaling, excessive redness, foreign bodies.

Inspect tympanic membrane

■ *Landmarks*

Vary light direction to observe entire membrane and annulus.	**EXPECTED:** Visible umbo, handle of malleus, and light reflex. **UNEXPECTED:** Perforations, landmarks not visible.

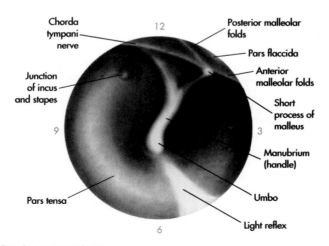

From Barkauskas et al, 1998.

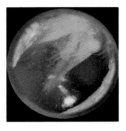

From Barkauskas et al, 1998.

TECHNIQUE	FINDINGS
■ *Color*	**EXPECTED:** Translucent, pearly gray. **UNEXPECTED:** Amber, yellow, blue, deep red, chalky white, dull, white flecks, or dense white plaques; air bubbles or fluid level.
■ *Contour*	**EXPECTED:** Slightly conical with concavity at umbo. **UNEXPECTED:** Bulging (more conical, usually with loss of bony landmarks and distorted light reflex) or retracted (more concave, usually with accentuated bony landmarks and distorted light reflex).
■ *Mobility* Seal canal with speculum, and *gently* apply positive (squeeze) and negative (release) pressure with pneumatic attachment.	**EXPECTED:** Movement in and out. **UNEXPECTED:** No movement.
Assess hearing	
■ *Questions during history*	**EXPECTED:** Responds to questions appropriately. **UNEXPECTED:** Excessive requests for repetition. Speech with monotonous tone and erratic volume.

TECHNIQUE	FINDINGS

- *Whispered voice*
  Have patient mask hearing in one ear by moving a finger rapidly up and down in ear canal. Stand 1 to 2 feet from other ear and softly whisper 1 to 2 syllable words. Repeat with untested ear.

  EXPECTED: Patient repeats words correctly at least 50% of the time.
  UNEXPECTED: Patient unable to repeat whispered words.

- *Ticking watch*
  Have patient mask hearing in one ear. Move watch toward other ear from about 5 inches. Repeat with untested ear.

  EXPECTED: Patient hears ticking at distance common for most people.
  UNEXPECTED: Patient unable to hear watch tick.

- *Weber test*
  Place base of vibrating tuning fork on midline vertex of head. Repeat with one ear occluded.

  EXPECTED: Sound heard equally in both ears (unoccluded). Sound heard better in occluded ear.
  UNEXPECTED: See the table on p. 80.

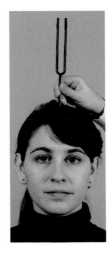

Weber test

Interpretation of Tuning Fork Tests

TEST	EXPECTED FINDINGS	CONDUCTIVE HEARING LOSS	SENSORINEURAL HEARING LOSS
Weber	No lateralization, but will lateralize to ear occluded by patient	Lateralization to deaf ear unless sensorineural loss	Lateralization to better ear unless conductive loss
Rinne	Air conduction heard longer than bone conduction by 2:1 ratio (*Rinne positive*)	Bone conduction heard longer than air conduction in affected ear (*Rinne negative*)	Air conduction heard longer than bone conduction in affected ear, but less than 2:1 ratio
Schwabach	Examiner hears equally as long as the patient	Patient hears longer than the examiner	Examiner hears longer than the patient

TECHNIQUE	FINDINGS

■ *Rinne test*

Place base of vibrating tuning fork against mastoid bone and note seconds until sound is no longer heard, then quickly move fork 1 to 2 cm ($^1/_2$ to 1 in) from auditory canal and note seconds until sound is no longer heard. Repeat with other ear.

EXPECTED: Measurement of air-conducted sound twice as long as measurement of bone-conducted sound.

UNEXPECTED: See the table on p. 80.

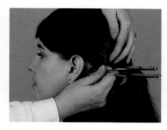 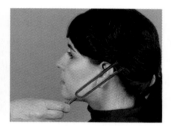

Rinne test

■ *Schwabach test*

Alternately place vibrating tuning fork against patient's mastoid and your mastoid until one of you no longer hears sound.

EXPECTED: Sound heard equal length of time by patient and examiner.

UNEXPECTED: See table on p. 80.

Nose and Sinuses

Inspect external nose

■ *Shape/size*

EXPECTED: Smooth. Columella directly midline, width is not greater than diameter of naris.

UNEXPECTED: Swelling or depression of nasal bridge. Transverse crease at junction of nose cartilage and bone.

TECHNIQUE	FINDINGS
■ *Color*	**EXPECTED:** Conforms to face color.
■ *Nares*	**EXPECTED:** Oval. Symmetrically positioned.
	UNEXPECTED: Asymmetry, discharge, flaring, narrowing.

Palpate ridge and soft tissues of nose

	EXPECTED: Firm and stable structures.
	UNEXPECTED: Displacement of bone and cartilage, tenderness, or masses.

Evaluate patency of nares

Occlude one naris with finger on side of nose and ask patient to breathe through nose. Repeat with other naris.	**EXPECTED:** Noiseless, easy breathing.
	UNEXPECTED: Noisy breathing; occlusion.

Inspect nasal mucosa and nasal septum

Use nasal speculum and strong light. Do no overdilate naris or touch septum.	
■ *Color*	**EXPECTED:** Mucosa deep pink and glistening. Turbinates same color as surrounding area.
	UNEXPECTED: Increased redness of mucosa or localized redness and swelling in vestibule. Turbinates bluish gray or pale pink.
■ *Shape*	**EXPECTED:** Septum close to midline and fairly straight, thicker anteriorly than posteriorly. Inferior and middle turbinates visible.

TECHNIQUE	FINDINGS

UNEXPECTED: Asymmetry of posterior nasal cavities, septal deviation.

- *Condition*

EXPECTED: Possibly a film of clear discharge on septum. Possibly hairs in vestibule. Turbinates firm.

UNEXPECTED: Discharge, bleeding, crusting, masses, or lesions. Swollen, boggy turbinates. Perforated septum. Polyps.

Inspect frontal and maxillary sinus area.

UNEXPECTED: Swelling.

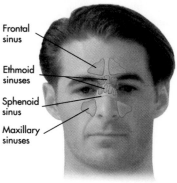

Frontal sinus

Ethmoid sinuses

Sphenoid sinus

Maxillary sinuses

Palpate frontal and maxillary sinuses

Press thumbs up under bony brow on each side of nose. Palpate with thumbs or index or middle fingers under zygomatic processes.

EXPECTED: Nontender on palpation.

UNEXPECTED: Tenderness, swelling, or pain.

TECHNIQUE	FINDINGS

Percuss frontal and maxillary sinuses

Lightly tap directly over each sinus with index finger.

EXPECTED: Hollow tone elicited.
UNEXPECTED: Tenderness, swelling, or pain.

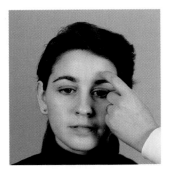
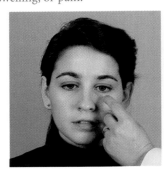

Mouth

Inspect and palpate lips with mouth closed

Have patient remove lipstick (if applicable).

- *Symmetry*

EXPECTED: Symmetric vertically and horizontally at rest and moving.
UNEXPECTED: Asymmetric.

- *Color*

EXPECTED: Pink, distinct border between lips and facial skin.
UNEXPECTED: Pallor, circumoral pallor, bluish purple, or cherry red.

- *Condition*

EXPECTED: Smooth.
UNEXPECTED: Swelling, angioedema; cheilosis; lesions; plaques; vesicles; nodules, ulcerations; or round, oval, or irregular bluish grey macules.

TECHNIQUE	FINDINGS

Inspect teeth

■ *Occlusion*
Have patient clench teeth and smile with lips spread.

EXPECTED: Upper molars resting directly on lower molars. Upper incisors slightly overriding lower incisors.
UNEXPECTED: Malocclusion.

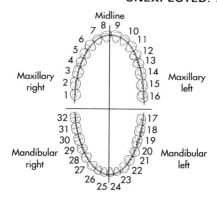

From Miyasaki-Ching, 1997.

■ *Color*

EXPECTED: Ivory, stained yellow or brown.
UNEXPECTED: Discolorations may indicate caries.

■ *Condition*

EXPECTED: 32 teeth.
UNEXPECTED: Caries and loose or missing teeth.

Inspect buccal mucosa

Have patient remove any dental appliances and then partially open mouth. Use tongue blade and bright light to assess.

■ *Color*

EXPECTED: Pinkish red.
UNEXPECTED: Deeply pigmented. Whitish or pinkish scars.

TECHNIQUE	FINDINGS

■ *Condition*

EXPECTED: Smooth and moist. Whitish yellow or whitish pink Stensen duct. Fordyce spots.
UNEXPECTED: Red spot at opening of Stensen duct. Ulcers.

Inspect and palpate gingiva

Use gloves to palpate.

■ *Color*

EXPECTED: Slightly stippled and pink.
UNEXPECTED: Blue-black line about 1 mm from gum margin.

■ *Condition*

EXPECTED: Clearly defined, tight margin at each tooth.
UNEXPECTED: Inflammation, swelling, bleeding, or lesions under dentures or on gingiva; induration, thickening, masses, or tenderness. Enlarged crevices between teeth and gum margins. Pockets containing debris at tooth margins.

Inspect tongue

■ *Size/symmetry*

EXPECTED: Midline.
UNEXPECTED: Atrophied, deviation to one side.

■ *Color*

EXPECTED: Dull red.

■ *Dorsum surface*

Have patient extend tongue and hold extended.

EXPECTED: Moist and glistening. Anterior: smooth yet roughened surface with papillae and small fissures. Posterior: smooth, slightly uneven or rugated surface with thinner mucosa than anterior. Possibly geographic.

TECHNIQUE	FINDINGS

UNEXPECTED: Smooth, red, and slick; hairy; swollen; coated; ulcerated. fasciculations; or limitation of movement.

- *Ventral surface and floor of mouth*
Have patient touch tip of tongue to palate behind upper incisors.

EXPECTED: Ventral surface pink and smooth with large veins between frenulum and fimbriated folds. Wharton ducts apparent on each side of frenulum.
UNEXPECTED: Difficulty touching hard palate. Swelling, varicosities.

- *Lateral borders*
Wrap tongue with gauze and pull to each side. Scrape white or red margins to remove food particles.

UNEXPECTED: Leukoplakia or other fixed abnormality.

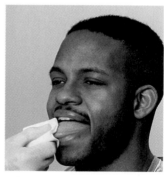

Palpate tongue and floor of mouth

EXPECTED: Smooth and even.
UNEXPECTED: Lumps, nodules, induration, ulcerations, or thickened white patches.

TECHNIQUE	FINDINGS

Inspect palate and uvula

Have patient tilt head back.

■ *Color and landmarks*

EXPECTED: Hard palate (whitish and dome-shaped with transverse rugae) contiguous with pinker soft palate. Bony protuberance of hard palate at midline (torus palatinus).
UNEXPECTED: Nodule on palate, not at midline.

■ *Movement*
Ask patient to say, "Ah" while observing soft palate. (Depress tongue if necessary.)

EXPECTED: Soft palate rises symmetrically, with uvula remaining in midline.
UNEXPECTED: Failure to rise bilaterally. Uvula deviation. Bifid uvula.

Inspect oropharynx

Depress tongue with tongue blade.

■ *Tonsils*

EXPECTED: Tonsils, if present, blend into pink color of pharynx. Possibly crypts in tonsils where cellular debris and food particles collect.
UNEXPECTED: Tonsils projecting beyond limits of tonsillar pillars. Tonsils red, enlarged, and covered with exudate.

■ *Posterior wall of pharynx*

EXPECTED: Smooth, glistening, pink mucosa with some small, irregular spots of lymphatic tissue and small blood vessels.

TECHNIQUE	FINDINGS
	UNEXPECTED: Red bulge adjacent to tonsil extending beyond midline. Yellowish mucoid film in pharynx. Grayish membrane.
Elicit gag reflex	
Touch posterior wall of pharynx on each side	**EXPECTED:** Bilateral response.
	UNEXPECTED: Unequal response or no response.

AIDS TO DIFFERENTIAL DIAGNOSIS

ABNORMALITY	DESCRIPTION
Bacterial otitis media	See table on p. 90.
Otitis media with effusion (serous otitis media)	See table on p. 90.
Sinusitis	Fever, headache, local tenderness, pain, swelling of skin overlying involved sinus, and copious purulent nasal discharge.
Tonsillitis	Sore throat, referred pain to ears, dysphagia, fever, fetid breath, and malaise. Tonsils are red and swollen. Tonsils covered with purulent exudate. May be studded with yellow follicles. Enlarged anterior cervical lymph nodes.
Peritonsillar abscess	Dysphagia, drooling, severe sore throat with pain radiating to ear, muffled voice, and fever. Tonsil, tonsillar pillar, and adjacent soft palate are red and swollen. Tonsil may appear pushed forward or backward, possibly displacing uvula.

Differentiating Between Otitis Externa, Bacterial Otitis Media, and Otitis Media With Effusion

SIGNS AND SYMPTOMS	OTITIS EXTERNA	BACTERIAL OTITIS MEDIA	OTITIS MEDIA WITH EFFUSION
Initial symptoms	Itching in ear canal	Fever, irritability, feeling of blockage, tugging earlobe	Sticking or cracking sound on yawning or swallowing
Pain	Intense with movement of pinna, chewing	Deep-seated earache	Uncommon; feeling of fullness
Discharge	Watery, then purulent and thick, mixed with pus and epithelial cells; musty, foul-smelling	Only if tympanic membrane ruptures; foul-smelling	Uncommon
Hearing	Conductive loss caused by exudate and swelling of ear canal	Conductive loss as middle ear fills with pus	Conductive loss as middle ear fills with fluid
Inspection	Canal is red, edematous; tympanic membrane obscured	Tympanic membrane may be red, thickened, bulging; impaired movement	Tympanic membrane is retracted, yellowish; impaired mobility; air level and/or bubbles

ABNORMALITY	DESCRIPTION
Nasal polyps	Boggy mucosa, rounded, elongated, and extending into nasal cavity.
Periodontal disease	Easily bleeding, swollen gums, enlarged crevices between teeth and gum margins.
Malocclusion	Teeth malpositioned, upper and lower molars not aligned, line of occlusion is incorrect.
Dental caries	Discolorations on the crown.

PEDIATRIC VARIATIONS

EXAMINATION

TECHNIQUE	FINDINGS

Ears

Inspect tympanic membrane

In children, pull auricle downward and back.	**EXPECTED:** The tympanic membrane may be red from crying. If red from crying, it will be mobile.

Assess hearing

■ *Evaluate response to auditory stimuli.*	**EXPECTED:** For infants, see table below.

Sequences of Expected Hearing Response in Infants	
AGE	RESPONSE
Birth to 3 months	Startle reflex, crying, cessation of breathing or movement in response to sudden noise; quiets to parent's voice
4 to 6 months	Turns head toward source of sound, but may not always recognize location of sound; responds to parent's voice; enjoys sound-producing toys
6 to 10 months	Responds to own name, telephone ringing, and person's voice, even if not loud; begins localizing sounds above and below, turns head 45 degrees toward sound
10 to 12 months	Recognizes and localizes source of sound; imitates simple words and sounds

TECHNIQUE	FINDINGS

■ *Whispered voice*

EXPECTED: In young children, patient should turn toward sound consistently.

Nose and Sinuses
Evaluate patency of nares

With the infant's mouth closed, or with infant sucking on bottle or pacifier, occlude one naris and then the other. Observe the respiratory pattern.

EXPECTED: Obligatory nose breathing until 2 to 3 months of age.

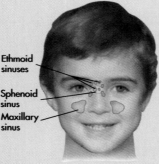

Ethmoid sinuses

Sphenoid sinus

Maxillary sinus

Mouth
Inspect and palpate lips with mouth closed

EXPECTED: In infants, sucking calluses, drooling from age 6 weeks to 6 months.
UNEXPECTED: Drooling persistent after age 12 months.

Inspect teeth

■ *Color*

EXPECTED: 0 to 20 teeth until age 6 years. Permanent teeth start erupting around age 6.

Inspect buccal mucosa

■ *Condition*

EXPECTED: In infants, nonadherent white patches (milk).

TECHNIQUE	FINDINGS
	UNEXPECTED: In infants, adherent white patches.
Inspect and palpate gingiva	
■ *Condition*	**EXPECTED:** In infants, Epstein pearls.

AIDS TO DIFFERENTIAL DIAGNOSIS

ABNORMALITY	DESCRIPTION
Epiglottitis	High fever, croupy cough, sore throat, drooling, difficulty breathing.

SAMPLE DOCUMENTATION

Ears. Auricles in alignment, lobes are pierced without masses, lesions, or tenderness. Canals unobstructed and coated with minimal amount of brown cerumen. Tympanic membranes are pearly gray, noninjected, intact, with bony landmarks and light reflex visualized bilaterally. No evidence of fluid or retraction.

Conversational hearing appropriate. Able to hear whispered voice. Weber—lateralizes equally to both ears, Rinne—air conduction greater than bone conduction bilaterally.

Nose. No discharge or polyps, mucosa pink and moist, septum midline, patent bilaterally. No edema over frontal or maxillary sinuses. No sinus tenderness to palpation. Correctly identifies mint, banana, and ammonia odors.

Mouth. Buccal mucosa pink and moist without lesions; 26 teeth present in various states of repair. Lower second molars absent bilaterally. Gingiva pink and firm. Tongue midline with no tremors or fasciculation.

Pharynx. Clear without erythema, tonsils 1+ without exudates. Uvula rises evenly and gag reflex is intact. No hoarseness. Patient identifies tastes of salt and sugar.

CLINICAL AND
REFERENCE NOTES

CHAPTER 9

CHEST AND LUNGS

EQUIPMENT

- Drape
- Marking pencil
- Ruler and tape measure
- Stethoscope with bell and diaphragm

EXAMINATION

Have patient sit, disrobed to waist.

TECHNIQUE	FINDINGS

Inspect front and back of chest

See thoracic landmarks.
- *Size/shape/symmetry*
- *Landmarks*

EXPECTED: Supernumerary nipples possible (but could be clue to other congenital abnormalities).

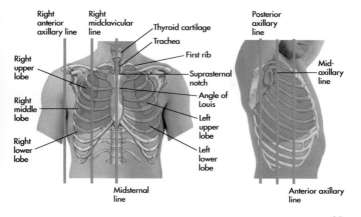

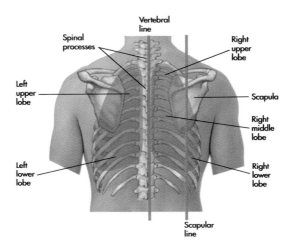

TECHNIQUE	FINDINGS
■ *Compare anteroposterior diameter with transverse diameter*	**EXPECTED:** Ribs prominent, clavicles prominent superiorly, and sternum usually flat and free of abundance of overlying tissue. Chest somewhat asymmetric. Anteroposterior diameter often one-half transverse diameter. **UNEXPECTED:** Barrel chest, posterior or lateral deviation, pigeon chest, or funnel chest.
■ *Assess nails, lips, and nares*	**UNEXPECTED:** Clubbed fingernails, pursed lips, flared alae nasi.
■ *Color* Assess skin, lips, and nails.	**UNEXPECTED:** Superficial venous patterns. Cyanosis or pallor of lips or nails.
■ *Breath*	**UNEXPECTED:** Malodorous.

TECHNIQUE	FINDINGS

Evaluate respirations

■ *Rhythm or pattern and rate*
See patterns of respiration in the figure below.

EXPECTED: Breathing easy, regular, and without distress. Pattern even. Rate 12 to 20 respirations/minute. Ratio of respirations to heartbeats about 1:4.

UNEXPECTED: Dyspnea, orthopnea, paroxysmal nocturnal dyspnea, platypnea, tachypnea, and hypopnea. Use of accessory muscles, retractions.

Normal	Regular and comfortable at a rate of 12-20 per minute	Air trapping	Increasing difficulty in getting breath out
Bradypnea	Slower than 12 breaths per minute	Cheyne-Stokes	Varying periods of increasing depth interspersed with apnea
Tachypnea	Faster than 20 breaths per minute	Kussmaul	Rapid, deep, labored
Hyperventilation (hyperpnea)	Faster than 20 breaths per minute, deep breathing	Biot	Irregularly interspersed periods of apnea in a disorganized sequence of breaths
Sighing	Frequently interspersed deeper breath	Ataxic	Significant disorganization with irregular and varying depths of respiration

TECHNIQUE	FINDINGS

■ *Inspiration/expiration ratio*   **UNEXPECTED:** Air trapping, prolonged expiration.

Inspect chest movement with breathing

■ *Symmetry*   **EXPECTED:** Chest expansion bilaterally symmetric.
UNEXPECTED: Asymmetry. Unilateral or bilateral bulging. Bulging on expiration.

Listen to respiration sounds audible without stethoscope

EXPECTED: Generally bronchovesicular.
UNEXPECTED: Crepitus, stridor, wheezes.

Palpate thoracic muscles and skeleton

■ *Symmetry/condition*   **EXPECTED:** Bilateral symmetry. Some elasticity of rib cage, but sternum and xiphoid relatively inflexible and thoracic spine rigid.
UNEXPECTED: Pulsations, tenderness, bulges, depressions, unusual movement, and unusual positions.

TECHNIQUE	**FINDINGS**

■ *Thoracic expansion*
Stand behind patient. Place palms in light contact with posterolateral surfaces and thumbs along spinal processes at tenth rib, as shown in the figure at right. Watch thumb divergence during quiet and deep breathing. Face patient; place thumbs along costal margin and xiphoid process with palms touching anterolateral chest. Watch thumb divergence during quiet and deep breathing.

EXPECTED: Symmetric expansion.
UNEXPECTED: Asymmetric expansion.

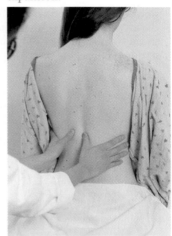

■ *Sensations*

EXPECTED: Nontender sensations.
UNEXPECTED: Crepitus or grating vibration.

■ *Tactile fremitus*
Ask patient to recite numbers or words while systematically palpating chest with palmar surfaces of fingers or ulnar aspect of clenched fist, using firm, light touch. Assess each area, front to back, side to side, and lung apices. Compare sides.

EXPECTED: Great variability.
UNEXPECTED: Decreased or absent fremitus; increased fremitus (coarser, rougher); or gentle, more tremulous fremitus; variation between similar positions on right and left thorax.

TECHNIQUE	FINDINGS

Note position of trachea

Using an index finger or thumbs, palpate gently from suprasternal notch along upper edges of each clavicle and in spaces above, to inner borders of sternocleidomastoid muscles.

EXPECTED: Spaces equal side to side. Trachea midline directly above suprasternal notch. Possible slight deviation to right.
UNEXPECTED: Significant deviation or tug. Pulsations.

Perform direct or indirect percussion on chest

Percuss directly or indirectly, as shown in the figures below. Compare all areas bilaterally, following a sequence such as shown in the top figures on p. 101.

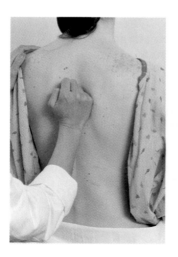
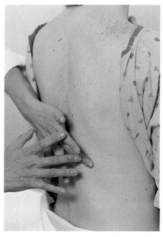

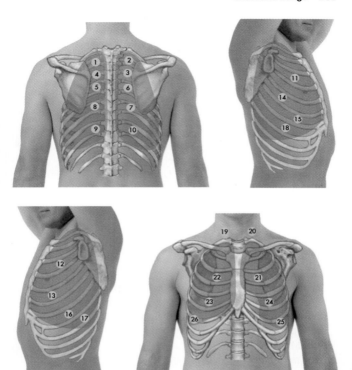

Percussion Tones Heard Over the Chest				
TYPE OF TONE	**INTENSITY**	**PITCH**	**DURATION**	**QUALITY**
Resonant	Loud	Low	Long	Hollow
Flat	Soft	High	Short	Extremely dull
Dull	Medium	Medium-high	Medium	Thudlike
Tympanic	Loud	High	Medium	Drumlike
Hyperresonant*	Very loud	Very low	Longer	Booming

From Thompson et al, 1997.

*Hyperresonance is an unexpected sound in adults. It represents air trapping, which occurs in obstructive lung diseases.

TECHNIQUE	FINDINGS

See the table on p. 101 for common tones, intensity, pitch, duration, and quality.

■ *Thorax*

Have patient sit with head bent and arms folded in front while percussing posterior thorax, then with arms raised overhead while percussing lateral and anterior chest. Percuss at 4 to 5 cm intervals over intercostal spaces, moving superior to inferior, medial to lateral.

EXPECTED: Resonance over all areas of lungs, dull over heart and liver, spleen, areas of thorax.
UNEXPECTED: Hyperresonance, dullness, or flatness.

■ *Diaphragmatic excursion*

Ask patient to breathe deeply and hold breath. Percuss along scapular line on one side until tone changes from resonant to dull. Mark skin. Allow patient to breathe normally, then repeat on other side. Have patient take several breaths, then exhale as much as possible and hold. On each side, percuss up from mark to change from dull to resonant. Tell patient to resume breathing comfortably. Measure excursion distance.

EXPECTED: 3 to 5 cm. Higher on right than left.
UNEXPECTED: Limited descent.

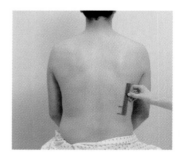

TECHNIQUE	FINDINGS

Auscultate chest with stethoscope diaphragm, apex to base

■ *Intensity, pitch, duration, and quality of breath sounds*
Have patient breathe slowly and deeply through mouth. Follow set auscultation sequence, holding stethoscope as shown in the figure at right. Ask patient to sit upright (1) with head bent and arms folded in front while auscultating posterior thorax, (2) with arms raised overhead while auscultating lateral chest, and (3) with arms down and shoulders back while auscultating anterior chest.

EXPECTED: See expected breath sounds in the table below.
UNEXPECTED: Amphoric or cavernous breathing. Sounds difficult to hear or absent. Crackles, rhonchi, wheezes, or pleural friction rub, as described in the table on p. 104.

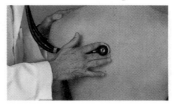

Characteristics of Expected Breath Sounds		
SOUND	CHARACTERISTICS	FINDINGS
Vesicular	Heard over most of lung fields; low pitch; soft and short expirations; will be accentuated in a thin person or a child and diminished in the overweight or very muscular patient	
Bronchovesicular	Heard over main bronchus area and over upper right posterior lung field; medium pitch; expiration equals inspiration	
Bronchial tracheal (tubular)	Heard only over trachea; high pitch; loud and long expirations, often somewhat longer than inspiration	

Modified from Thompson et al, 1997.

Adventitious Breath Sounds

Fine crackles: high-pitched, discrete, discontinuous crackling sounds heard during the end of inspiration; not cleared by cough

Medium crackles: lower, more moist sound heard during the midstage of inspiration, not cleared by a cough

Coarse crackles: loud, bubbly noise heard during inspiration; not cleared by a cough

Rhonchi (sonorous wheeze): loud, low, coarse sounds, like a snore, most often heard continuously during inspiration or expiration; coughing may clear sound (usually means mucus accumulation in trachea or large bronchi)

Wheeze (sibilant wheeze): musical noise sounding like a squeak; most often heard continuously during inspiration or expiration; usually louder during expiration

Pleural friction rub: dry, rubbing, or grating sound, usually caused by inflammation of pleural surfaces; heard during inspiration or expiration; loudest over lower lateral anterior surface

Modified from Thompson et al, 1997.

TECHNIQUE	FINDINGS
Listen during inspiration and expiration. Auscultate downward from apex to base at intervals of several centimeters, making side-to-side comparisons. ■ *Vocal resonance* Ask patient to recite numbers or words.	**EXPECTED:** Muffled and indistinct sounds. **UNEXPECTED:** Bronchophony, whispered pectoriloquy, or egophony.

AIDS TO DIFFERENTIAL DIAGNOSIS

ABNORMALITY	SYMPTOM
Lung cancer	Cough, wheezing, emphysema, atelectasis, pneumonitis, and hemoptysis. Possible sputum.
Infections	Sputum production (see the table on p. 107).
Cough-producing conditions	See the box on p. 106.
Asthma	Cough, wheezing, respiratory distress, tachypnea, pallor to cyanosis; possible decreased breath sounds; possibly allergy or exercise induced.
Chronic obstructive pulmonary disease	Barrel chest, hyperresonance to percussion, sputum production, cough, prolonged expiration, amphoric breathing.

Assessing Cough

Coughs are a common symptom of a respiratory problem. They are usually preceded by a deep inspiration; this is followed by closure of the glottis, relaxation of the diaphragm, and then a sudden, spasmodic expiration, forcing a sudden opening of the glottis. The causes may be related to localized or more general insults at any point in the respiratory tract. Coughs may be voluntary, but they are usually reflexive responses to an irritant such as a foreign body (microscopic or larger), an infectious agent, or a mass of any sort compressing the respiratory tree. They may also be a clue to an anxiety state.

Describe a cough according to its moisture, frequency, regularity, pitch and loudness, and quality. The type of cough may offer some clue to the cause. Although a cough may not have a serious cause, it should not be ignored.

Dry or moist. A moist cough may be caused by infection and can be accompanied by sputum production. A dry cough can have a variety of causes (for example, cardiac problems, allergies, or AIDS), which may be indicated by the quality of its sound.

Onset. An acute onset, particularly with fever, suggests infection; in the absence of fever, a foreign body or inhaled irritants are additional possible causes.

Frequency of occurrence. Note whether the cough is seldom or often present. An infrequent cough may result from allergens or environmental insults.

Regularity. A regular, paroxysmal cough is heard in pertussis. An irregularly occurring cough may have a variety of causes, such as smoking, early congestive heart failure, an inspired foreign body or irritant, or a tumor within or compressing the bronchial tree.

Pitch and loudness. A cough may be loud and high pitched or quiet and relatively low pitched.

Postural influences. A cough may occur soon after a person has reclined or assumed an erect position (for example, with a nasal drip or pooling of secretions in the upper airway).

Quality. A dry cough may sound brassy if it is caused by compression of the respiratory tree (as by a tumor) or hoarse if it is caused by croup. Pertussis produces an inspiratory "whoop" at the end of a paroxysm of coughing.

Assessing Sputum	
CAUSE	POSSIBLE SPUTUM CHARACTERISTICS
Bacterial infection	Yellow, green, rust-colored (blood mixed with yellow sputum), clear, or transparent; purulent; blood streaked; mucoid, viscid
Viral infection	Mucoid, viscid; blood streaked (not common)
Chronic infectious disease	All of the above; particularly abundant in the early morning; slight, intermittent blood streaking; occasionally large amounts of blood
Carcinoma	Slight, persistent blood streaking
Infarction	Blood clotted; large amounts of blood
Tuberculous cavity	Large amounts of blood

PEDIATRIC VARIATIONS

EXAMINATION

TECHNIQUE	FINDINGS

Inspect front and back of chest

- *Compare anteroposterior diameter with transverse diameter*

EXPECTED: An infant's chest is expected to measure 2 to 3 cm less than head circumference.

Evaluate respirations

- *Rhythm or pattern and rate*

EXPECTED:

AGE	RESPIRATIONS PER MINUTE
Newborn	30-80
1 year	20-40
3 years	20-30
6 years	16-22
10 years	16-20
17 years	12-20

TECHNIQUE	FINDINGS

Perform direct or indirect percussion on chest

- *Thorax*

EXPECTED: Hyperresonance may be heard in children.

Auscultate chest with stethoscope diaphragm, apex to base

- *Intensity, pitch, duration, and quality of breath sounds*

EXPECTED: In infants and children, expect transmitted breath sounds throughout the chest. Vesicular sound will be accentuated in a child. Absent or diminished breath sounds are harder to detect.

SAMPLE DOCUMENTATION

Minimal increase in the anteroposterior diameter of chest, without kyphosis or other distortion. Thoracic expansion symmetric. Respiration rapid and somewhat labored, not accompanied by retractions or stridor. On palpation, trachea in midline without tug; no friction rubs or tenderness over ribs or other bony prominence. Over the left base posteriorly, tactile fremitus is diminished; percussion note was dull; on auscultation, crackles were heard that did not clear with cough; breath sounds diminished. Remainder of lung fields clear and free of adventitious sounds, with resonant percussion tones. On percussion the diaphragm descended 3 cm bilaterally at midscapular line.

CHAPTER 10

HEART AND BLOOD VESSELS

EQUIPMENT

- Tangential light source
- Marking pencil
- Stethoscope with bell and diaphragm
- Sphygmomanometer
- Centimeter ruler

EXAMINATION

TECHNIQUE	FINDINGS

Heart

Inspect precordium

Have patient supine and keep the light source tangential.

- *Apical impulse*

EXPECTED: Visible about midclavicular line in fifth left intercostal space. Sometimes only visible with patient sitting.
UNEXPECTED: Visible in more than one intercostal space; exaggerated lifts or heaves.

TECHNIQUE	FINDINGS

Palpate precordium and carotid artery

- *Apical impulse*
  Have patient supine. With hands *warm,* gently feel precordium, using proximal halves of the fingers held together or whole hand. As shown in the figure at right, methodically move from apex to left sternal border, base, right sternal border, epigastrium, and axillae. Locate the sensation in terms of its intercostal space and relationship to midsternal, midclavicular, and axillary lines.

EXPECTED: Gentle, brief impulse, palpable within radius of 1 cm or less, although often not felt.
UNEXPECTED: Heave or lift, loss of thrust, displacement to right or left; or thrill.

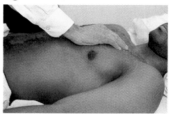

- *Carotid artery*
  Use other hand to palpate carotid artery, as shown in the figure at right, to describe carotid pulse in relation to cardiac cycle.

EXPECTED: Carotid pulse and first heart sound (S_1) practically synchronous.
UNEXPECTED: Asynchrony.

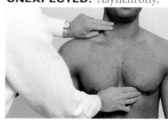

TECHNIQUE	FINDINGS

Percuss precordium (optional)

Begin by tapping at anterior axillary line, moving medially along intercostal spaces toward sternal borders until tone changes from resonance to dullness. Mark skin with pencil.

EXPECTED: No change in tone before right sternal border; on left, loss of resonance generally close to point of maximal impulse at fifth intercostal space. Loss of resonance may outline the left border of heart at second to fifth intercostal spaces.

Auscultate in the five auscultatory areas

Make certain patient is warm and relaxed. Isolate each sound and each pause in the cycle, and then inch along with the stethoscope. Approach each of the five precordial areas shown in the figure on p. 112 systematically, base to apex or apex to base, using each of the positions shown in the figures at right. Use the diaphragm of the stethoscope first, with firm pressure, then the bell, with light pressure.

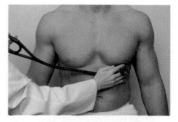

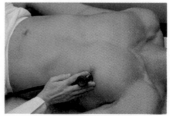

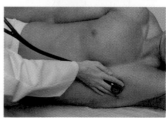

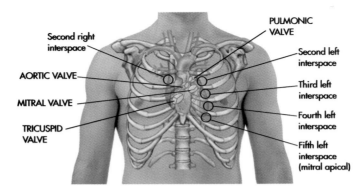

Label (left)	Label (right)
Second right interspace	PULMONIC VALVE
AORTIC VALVE	Second left interspace
MITRAL VALVE	Third left interspace
TRICUSPID VALVE	Fourth left interspace
	Fifth left interspace (mitral apical)

TECHNIQUE	FINDINGS
■ *Rate and rhythm* Assess overall rate and rhythm.	**EXPECTED:** Rate 60 to 90 beats/minute, regular rhythm. **UNEXPECTED:** Bradycardia, tachycardia, arrhythmia.
■ S_1 Ask patient to breathe comfortably, then hold breath in expiration. Listen for S_1 (best heard toward apex) while palpating carotid pulse. Note intensity, variations, effect of respiration, and splitting. Concentrate on systole, then diastole.	**EXPECTED:** S_1 usually heard as one sound and coincides with rise of carotid pulse. See the table on p. 113 and the figure on p. 114. **UNEXPECTED:** Extra sounds or murmurs.
■ S_2 Ask patient to breathe comfortably as you listen for S_2 (best heard in aortic and pulmonic areas) to become two components during inspiration. Ask patient to inhale and hold breath.	**EXPECTED:** S_2 to become two components during inspiration. S_2 to become an apparent single sound as breath exhaled. See the table on p. 113 and the figure on p. 114.

Heart Sounds According to Auscultatory Area

	AORTIC	PULMONIC	SECOND PULMONIC	MITRAL	TRICUSPID
Pitch	$S_1 < S_2$	$S_1 < S_2$	$S_1 < S_2$	$S_1 < S_2$	$S_1 < S_2$
Loudness	$S_1 < S_2$	$S_1 < S_2$	$S_1 < S_2$*	$S_1 > S_2$†	$S_1 > S_2$
Duration	$S_1 > S_2$	$S_1 > S_2$	$S_1 > S_2$	$S_1 > S_2$	$S_1 > S_2$
S_2 split	>Inhale	>Inhale	>Inhale	>Inhale‡	>Inhale
	<Exhale	<Exhale	<Exhale	<Exhale	<Exhale
A_2	Loudest	Loud	Decreased		
P_2	Decreased	Louder	Loudest		

*S_1 is relatively louder in second pulmonic area than in aortic area.
†S_1 may be louder in mitral area than in tricuspid area.
‡S_2 split may not be audible in mitral area if P_2 is inaudible.

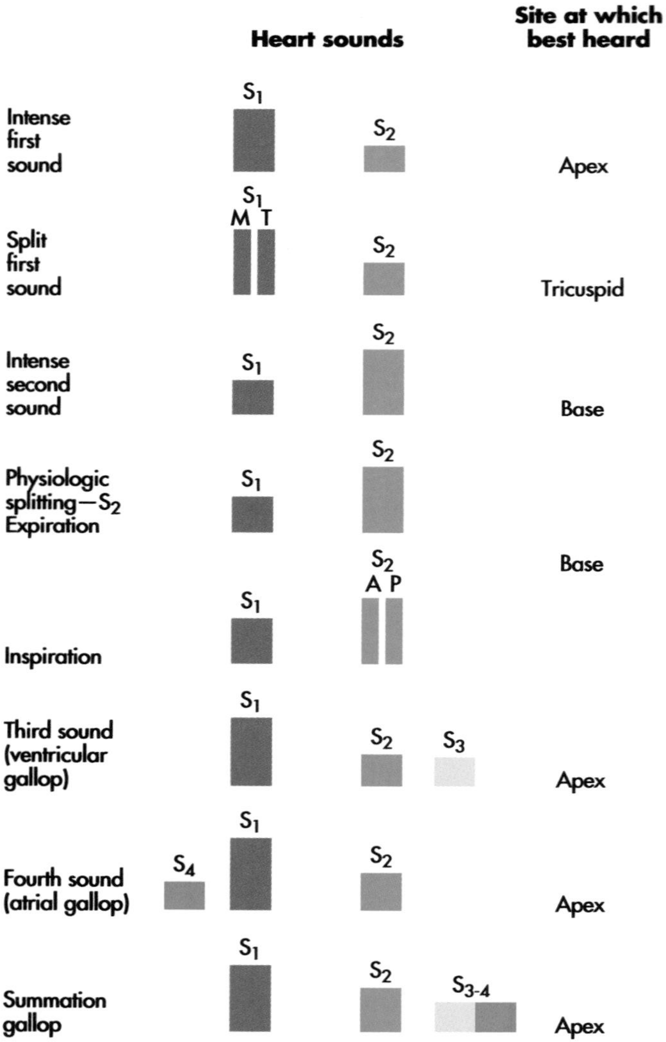

Heart sounds

Site at which best heard

Intense first sound	S_1 S_2	Apex
Split first sound	S_1 M T S_2	Tricuspid
Intense second sound	S_1 S_2	Base
Physiologic splitting—S_2 Expiration	S_1 S_2	Base
Inspiration	S_1 S_2 A P	
Third sound (ventricular gallop)	S_1 S_2 S_3	Apex
Fourth sound (atrial gallop)	S_4 S_1 S_2	Apex
Summation gallop	S_1 S_2 S_{3-4}	Apex

TECHNIQUE	FINDINGS

■ *Splitting*

EXPECTED: S_2 splitting—greatest at peak of inspiration—varying from easily heard to nondetectable.

■ *S_3 and S_4*
  If needed, ask patient to raise a leg to increase venous return or to grip your hand vigorously and repeatedly to increase arterial pressure

EXPECTED: Both S_3 and S_4 quiet and difficult to hear.
UNEXPECTED: Increased intensity (and ease of hearing) of either.

■ *Extra heart sounds*

UNEXPECTED: Extra heart sounds—snaps, clicks, friction rubs, and murmurs. See the table on p. 116 and the figure on p. 114.

Assess characteristics of murmurs

■ *Timing and duration, pitch, intensity, pattern, quality, location, radiation, respiratory phase variations*

See the table on p. 116.

Peripheral Arteries

Palpate arterial pulses in distal extremities

Palpate carotid, brachial, radial, femoral, popliteal, dorsalis pedis, and posterior tibial arteries, using distal pads of second and third fingers, as shown in the figures on p. 117.

Extra Heart Sounds

SOUND	DETECTION	DESCRIPTION
Increased S_3	Bell at apex; patient left lateral recumbent	Early diastole, low pitch
Increased S_4	Bell at apex; patient supine or semilateral	Late diastole or early systole, low pitch
Gallops	Bell at apex; patient supine or left lateral recumbent	Presystole, intense, easily heard
Mitral valve opening snap	Diaphragm medial to apex, may radiate to base; any position, second left intercostal	Early diastole briefly, before S_3; high pitch, sharp snap or click; not affected by respiration; easily confused with S_2
Ejection clicks	Diaphragm; patient sitting or supine	
Aortic valve	Apex, base in second right intercostal space	Early systole, intense, high pitch; radiates; not affected by respirations
Pulmonary valve	Second left intercostal space at sternal border	Early systole, less intense than aortic click; intensifies on expiration, decreases on inspiration
Pericardial friction rub	Widely heard, sound clearest toward apex	May occupy all of systole and diastole; intense, grating, machinelike; may have three components and obliterate heart sounds; if only one or two components, may sound like murmur

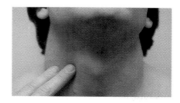

Carotid

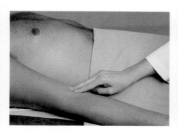

Brachial

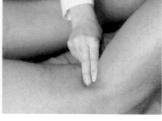

Radial

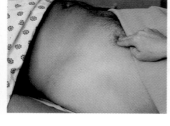

Femoral

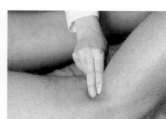

Popliteal

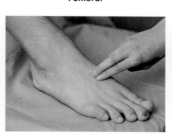

Dorsalis pedis

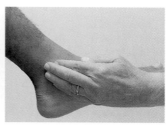

Posterior tibial

TECHNIQUE	FINDINGS
■ *Characteristics* Compare characteristics bilaterally, as well as between upper and lower extremities.	**EXPECTED:** Femoral pulse as strong as or stronger than radial pulse. **UNEXPECTED:** Femoral pulse weaker than radial pulse or absent, alternating pulse (pulsus alternans), pulsus bisferiens, bigeminal pulse (pulsus bigeminus), bounding pulse, labile pulse, paradoxic pulse (pulsus paradoxus), pulsus differens, tachycardia, trigeminal pulse (pulsus trigeminus), or water-hammer pulse (Corrigan pulse).
■ *Rate*	**EXPECTED:** 60 to 90 beats per minute.
■ *Rhythm*	**EXPECTED:** Regular. **UNEXPECTED:** Irregular, either in a pattern or patternless.
■ *Contour*	**EXPECTED:** Smooth, rounded, or domed shape.
■ *Amplitude*	**UNEXPECTED:** Bounding, full, diminished, or absent. Describe on scale of 0 to 4: 4 = bounding 3 = full, increased 2 = expected 1 = diminished 0 = absent, not palpable

Auscultate temporal carotid, subclavian, abdominal aorta, renal, iliac, and femoral arteries for bruits

You may at times need to ask patient to hold breath for a few heartbeats and auscultate with bell of stethoscope.	**UNEXPECTED:** Transmitted murmurs, bruits.

TECHNIQUE	FINDINGS

Assess for arterial occlusion and insufficiency

- *Site*
  Assess for pain distal to possible occlusion.

  UNEXPECTED: Dull ache accompanied by fatigue and often crampiness; possible constant or excruciating pain. Weak, thready, or absent pulses; systolic bruits over arteries; loss of body warmth; localized pallor or cyanosis; delay in venous filling; or thin, atrophied skin, muscle atrophy, and loss of hair.

- *Degree of occlusion*
  Ask patient to lie supine. Elevate extremity and note degree of blanching, then ask patient to sit on edge of table or bed to lower extremity. Note time for maximal return of color when extremity is elevated.

  EXPECTED: Slight pallor on elevation and return to full color as soon as leg becomes dependent.
  UNEXPECTED: Delay of more than 2 seconds.

Measure blood pressure

Measure in both arms at least once. Patient's arm should be slightly flexed and comfortably supported on table, pillow, or your hand.

EXPECTED: 100 to 140 mm Hg systolic and 60 to 90 mm Hg second diastolic, with pulse pressure of 30 to 40 mm Hg (sometimes to 50 mm Hg). Reading between arms may vary by as much as 10 mm Hg; usually higher in right arm.
UNEXPECTED: Hypertension (see the table on p. 120).

Classification of Blood Pressure for Adults Age 18 and Older*			
CATEGORY	SYSTOLIC (MM HG)		DIASTOLIC (MM HG)
Optimal†	<120	and	<80
Normal	<130	and	<85
High-normal	130-139	or	85-89
Hypertension‡			
Stage 1	140-159	or	90-99
Stage 2	160-179	or	100-109
Stage 3	≥180	or	≥110

From NIH Publication No. 48-4080, November 1997.
*Not taking antihypertensive drugs and not acutely ill. When systolic and diastolic blood pressures fall into different categories, the higher category should be selected to classify the individual's blood pressure status. For example, 160/92 mm Hg should be classified as stage 2 hypertension, and 124/120 mm Hg should be classified as stage 3 hypertension. Isolated systolic hypertension is defined as SBP of 140 mm Hg or greater and DBP below 90 mm Hg and staged appropriately (e.g., 170/82 mm Hg is defined as stage 2 isolated systolic hypertension). In addition to classifying stages of hypertension on the basis of average blood pressure levels, clinicians should specify presence or absence of target organ disease and additional risk factors. This specificity is important for risk classification and treatment.
†Optimal blood pressure with respect to cardiovascular risk is below 120/80 mm Hg. However, unusually low readings should be evaluated for clinical significance.
‡Based on the average of two or more readings taken at each of two or more visits after an initial screening.

TECHNIQUE   **FINDINGS**

Peripheral Veins

Assess jugular venous pressure

Ask patient to recline at 45-degree angle. With tangential light, observe both jugular veins. As shown in the figure at right, use a centimeter ruler to measure vertical distance between the midaxillary line and highest level of jugular vein distention.

EXPECTED: Pressure of 9 cm water or less, bilaterally symmetric.
UNEXPECTED: Abnormal distention or distention on one side.

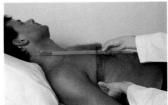

TECHNIQUE	FINDINGS

Assess for venous obstruction and insufficiency

Inspect extremities, with patient both standing and supine.

■ *Affected area*

UNEXPECTED: Constant pain with swelling and tenderness over muscles, engorgement of superficial veins, and cyanosis.

■ *Thrombosis*
Flex patient's knee slightly with one hand and with other, dorsiflex foot to test for Homans sign.

UNEXPECTED: Redness, thickening, and tenderness along superficial vein. Calf pain with test for Homans sign.

■ *Edema*
Press index finger over bony prominence of tibia or medial malleolus for several seconds.

UNEXPECTED: Orthostatic (pitting) edema; thickening and ulceration of skin possible. Grade edema 1+ to 4+ as follows:

1+ = Slight pitting, no visible distortion, disappears rapidly

2+ = Deeper than 1+ and disappears in 10 to 15 seconds

3+ = Noticeably deep and may last more than 1 minute, with dependent extremity full and swollen

4+ = Very deep and lasts 2 to 5 minutes, with grossly distorted dependent extremity

■ *Varicose veins*
If suspected, have patient stand on toes 10 times in succession.

EXPECTED: Pressure from toe standing disappears in seconds.
UNEXPECTED: Veins dilated and swollen; often tortuous when extremities are dependent and pressure does not quickly disappear.

TECHNIQUE	FINDINGS
If varicose veins are present, assess venous incompetence with Trendelenburg test: Ask patient to lie supine, lift leg above heart level until veins empty, then quickly lower leg.	**UNEXPECTED:** Rapid filling of veins.
Evaluate patency of deep veins with Perthes test: Ask patient to lie supine. Elevate extremity and occlude subcutaneous veins with tourniquet just above knee. Then ask patient to walk.	**UNEXPECTED:** Superficial veins fail to empty.
Evaluate direction of blood flow and presence of compensatory circulation: Put affected limb in dependent position, then empty or strip vein. Release pressure of one finger nearest the heart to assess blood flow; if necessary, repeat and release pressure of other finger.	**UNEXPECTED:** Stripped vessel fills before pressure is released, or blood refills entire vein when pressure is released.

AIDS TO DIFFERENTIAL DIAGNOSIS

ABNORMALITY	DESCRIPTION
Chest pain	See the box on p. 123.
Left ventricular hypertrophy	Vigorous sustained lift palpable during ventricular systole, sometimes over broader area than usual (by 2 cm or more). Displacement of apical impulse can be well lateral to midclavicular line and downward.

Chest Pain

TYPE OF CHEST PAIN	CHARACTERISTICS
Anginal	Substernal; provoked by effort, emotion, eating; relieved by rest and/or nitroglycerin
Pleural	Precipitated by breathing or coughing; usually described as sharp
Esophageal	Burning, substernal, occasional radiation to the shoulder; nocturnal occurrence, usually when lying flat; relief with food, antacids, sometimes nitroglycerin
From a peptic ulcer	Almost always infradiaphragmatic and epigastric; nocturnal occurrence and daytime attacks relieved by food; unrelated to activity
Biliary	Usually under right scapula, prolonged in duration; will trigger angina more often than mimic it
Arthritic/bursitis	Usually of hours-long duration; local tenderness and/or pain with movement
Cervical	Associated with injury; provoked by activity, persists after activity; painful on palpation and/or movement
Musculoskeletal (chest)	Intensified or provoked by movement, particularly twisting or costochondral bending; long lasting; often associated with local tenderness
Psychoneurotic	Associated with/after anxiety; poorly described, located in intramammary region

Modified from Samiy et al, 1987; Harvey et al, 1988.

ABNORMALITY	DESCRIPTION
Right ventricular hypertrophy	Lift along left sternal border in third and fourth left intercostal spaces accompanied by occasional systolic retraction at apex. Left ventricle displaced and turned posteriorly by enlarged right ventricle.

ABNORMALITY	DESCRIPTION
Congestive heart failure	Congestion in pulmonary or systemic circulation. Can be predominantly left- or right-sided and can develop gradually or suddenly with acute pulmonary edema.
Cor pulmonale	Left parasternal systolic lift and loud S_2 in the pulmonic region.
Myocardial infarction	Deep substernal or visceral pain, often radiating to jaw, neck, and left arm (although discomfort is sometimes mild); dysrhythmias; S_4 often present; heart sounds distant, with soft, systolic, blowing murmur; pulse possibly thready; varied blood pressure (although hypertension usual in early phases).
Myocarditis	Initial: fatigue, dyspnea, fever, and palpitations. Later: cardiac enlargement, murmur, gallop rhythms, tachycardia, dysrhythmias, and pulsus alternans.
Conduction disturbances	Transient weakness, fainting spells, or strokelike episodes.
Congenital defects	
Tetralogy of Fallot	Parasternal heave and precordial prominence. Cyanosis. Systolic ejection murmur heard over third intercostal space, sometimes radiating to left side of neck. Single S_2.
Ventricular septal defect	Arterial pulse small and jugular venous pulse unaffected. Regurgitation occurs through septal defect, resulting in holosystolic murmur that is frequently loud, coarse, high-pitched, and best

ABNORMALITY	DESCRIPTION
	heard along the left sternal border in the third to fifth intercostal spaces. Distinct lift often discernible along left sternal border and the apical area. Does not radiate to neck.
Coarctation of the aorta	Delay and/or palpable diminution in amplitude (not necessarily an absence) of femoral pulse when radial and femoral pulses are palpated simultaneously. Findings are same on right and left sides. Blood pressure in arms will be distinctly, even severely, higher than in legs. Possible systolic murmur audible over precordium and sometimes over back relative to area of coarctation. Adult x-ray examination may show notching of ribs and "3" sign in contour of left upper border of heart.
Patent ductus arteriosus	Neck vessels dilated and pulsate, and pulse pressure wide. Harsh, loud, continuous murmur with machinelike quality, heard at first to third intercostal spaces and lower sternal border. Murmur usually unaltered by postural change.
Atrial septal defect	Systolic ejection murmur—best heard over pulmonic area—that is diamond shaped, often loud, high in pitch, and harsh. May be accompanied by brief, rumbling, early diastolic murmur. Does not usually radiate beyond precordium. Systolic thrill

ABNORMALITY	DESCRIPTION
	may be felt over area of murmur along with palpable parasternal thrust. S_2 may be split fairly widely. Particularly significant with palpable thrust and occasional radiation through to back.
Dextrocardia and situs inversus	Altered clinical manifestations of disease (e.g., the substernal pressure of myocardial ischemia may be felt to the right of the precordium and may more often radiate to right arm).

Arterial/venous disorders

ABNORMALITY	DESCRIPTION
Arterial aneurysm	Pulsatile swelling along course of an artery—most commonly in the aorta, although intracranial, abdominal, renal, femoral, and popliteal arteries are also common. Thrill or bruit sometimes evident over aneurysm.
Venous thrombosis	Clinical findings in superficial vein include redness, thickening, and tenderness along involved segment. Deep vein thrombosis in femoral and pelvic circulations may be asymptomatic, but suggestive signs and symptoms include tenderness along iliac vessels and femoral canal, in popliteal space, and over deep calf veins, as well as slight swelling, minimal ankle edema, low-grade fever, and tachycardia.
Raynaud disease	Intermittent skin pallor or cyanosis, bilateral and lasting from minutes to hours. Skin

ABNORMALITY	DESCRIPTION
	over digits eventually appears smooth, shiny, and tight; ulcers may appear on tips of digits.
Mitral insufficiency	Usually silent and painless. Also occurs after infarction.
Atherosclerotic heart disease	Myocardial insufficiency, angina pectoris, dysrhythmias, and congestive heart failure.
Angina	Substernal pain or intense pressure radiating at times to neck, jaws, and arms, particularly the left arm. Often accompanied by shortness of breath, fatigue, diaphoresis, faintness, and syncope.

PEDIATRIC VARIATIONS

EXAMINATION

TECHNIQUE	FINDINGS

Heart

Assess characteristics of murmurs

- *Timing and duration, intensity, pattern, quality, location, radiation, respiratory phase variations* — In children it is necessary to distinguish innocent murmurs from organic murmurs caused by congenital defect or rheumatic fever.

Peripheral Arteries

Palpate arterial pulses in distal extremities

- *Rate*

EXPECTED:

AGE	BEATS PER MINUTE
Newborn	120-170
1 year	80-160
3 years	80-120
6 years	75-115
10 years	70-110

TECHNIQUE	FINDINGS

Auscultate arteries for bruits

EXPECTED: In children it is not unusual to hear a venous hum over internal jugular veins. There is usually no pathologic significance.

Measure blood pressure

When measuring an infant's blood pressure, use the flush technique if needed.

EXPECTED: Calculation of systolic blood pressure for children over 1 year of age can be estimated with the following formula:

$80 + (2 \times$ child's age in years)

Example: Calculation of expected systolic blood pressure of 5-year-old child:

$80 + (2 \times 5) = 90$

Although this calculation gives a figure below the expected mean, it is still considered within normal limits for a 5-year-old child.

UNEXPECTED: Hypertension (see tables on pp. 130-133).

AIDS TO DIFFERENTIAL DIAGNOSIS

ABNORMALITY	DESCRIPTION

Chest pain

Unlike in adults, chest pain in children and adolescents is seldom caused by a cardiac problem. It is very often difficult to find a cause, but trauma and exercise-induced asthma and the use of cocaine, even in a somewhat younger child as in the adolescent and adult, should be among the considerations.

SAMPLE DOCUMENTATION

Heart: No visible pulsations over precordium. The point of maximal impulse (PMI) palpable at the 5th ICS in the MCL, 1 cm in diameter. No lifts, heaves, or thrills felt on palpation. S_1 is crisp. Split S_2 increases with inspiration. No audible S_3, S_4, murmur, click, or rub.

Vessels: Neck veins not distended. Both A and V waves are visualized. The jugular venous pressure (JVP) is 4 cm water at 45 degrees. Arterial pulses equal and symmetric, testing on a scale of x/4.

	C	B	R	F	P	PT	DP
L	2+	2+	2+	2+	2+	2+	2+
R	2+	2+	2+	2+	2+	2+	2+

Vessels soft. No bruits are audible.

Extremities: No edema, skin, or nail changes. Superficial varicosities noted in both lower extremities. No areas of tenderness to palpation.

Blood Pressure Levels for the 90th and 95th Percentiles of Blood Pressure for Boys Aged 1 to 17 Years by Percentiles of Height

AGE, Y	BLOOD PRESSURE PERCENTILE*	SYSTOLIC BLOOD PRESSURE BY PERCENTILE OF HEIGHT, MM Hg†							DIASTOLIC BLOOD PRESSURE BY PERCENTILE OF HEIGHT, MM Hg†						
		5%	10%	25%	50%	75%	90%	95%	5%	10%	25%	50%	75%	90%	95%
1	90th	94	95	97	98	100	102	102	50	51	52	53	54	54	55
	95th	98	99	101	102	104	106	106	55	55	56	57	58	59	59
2	90th	98	99	100	102	104	105	106	55	55	56	57	58	59	59
	95th	101	102	104	106	108	109	110	59	59	60	61	62	63	63
3	90th	100	101	103	105	107	108	109	59	59	60	61	62	63	63
	95th	104	105	107	109	111	112	113	63	63	64	65	66	67	67
4	90th	102	103	105	107	109	110	111	62	62	63	64	65	66	66
	95th	106	107	109	111	113	114	115	66	67	67	68	69	70	71
5	90th	104	105	106	108	110	111	112	65	65	66	67	68	69	69
	95th	108	109	110	112	114	115	116	69	70	70	71	72	73	74
6	90th	105	106	108	110	111	113	114	67	68	69	70	70	71	72
	95th	109	110	112	114	115	117	117	72	72	73	74	75	76	76
7	90th	106	107	109	111	113	114	115	69	70	71	72	72	73	74
	95th	110	111	113	115	116	118	119	74	74	75	76	77	78	78
8	90th	107	108	110	112	114	115	116	71	71	72	73	74	75	75
	95th	111	112	114	116	118	119	120	75	76	76	77	78	79	80
9	90th	109	110	112	113	115	117	117	72	73	73	74	75	76	77

Age	Percentile	Systolic BP by height percentile†							Diastolic BP by height percentile†						
	95th	113	114	116	117	119	121	121	76	77	78	79	80	80	81
10	90th	110	112	113	115	117	118	119	73	74	74	75	76	77	78
10	95th	114	115	117	119	121	122	123	77	78	79	80	80	81	82
11	90th	112	113	115	117	119	120	121	74	74	75	76	77	78	78
11	95th	116	117	119	121	123	124	125	78	79	79	80	81	82	83
12	90th	115	116	117	119	121	123	123	75	75	76	77	78	78	79
12	95th	119	120	121	123	125	126	127	79	80	80	81	82	83	83
13	90th	117	118	120	122	124	125	126	75	76	76	77	78	79	80
13	95th	121	122	124	126	128	129	130	80	81	81	82	83	83	84
14	90th	120	121	123	125	126	128	128	76	77	77	78	79	80	80
14	95th	124	125	127	128	130	132	132	81	82	83	82	83	84	85
15	90th	123	124	125	127	129	131	131	77	78	78	79	80	81	81
15	95th	127	128	129	131	133	134	135	81	83	83	83	84	85	86
16	90th	125	126	128	130	132	133	134	79	80	80	81	82	82	83
16	95th	129	130	132	134	136	137	138	83	84	84	85	86	87	87
17	90th	128	129	131	133	134	136	136	81	81	82	83	84	85	85
17	95th	132	133	135	136	138	140	140	85	85	86	87	88	89	89

From Update on Task force report on high blood pressure in children, 1996.
*Blood pressure percentile was determined by a single measurement.
†Height percentile was determined by standard growth curves.

Blood Pressure Levels for the 90th and 95th Percentiles of Blood Pressure for Girls Aged 1 to 17 Years by Percentiles of Height

AGE, Y	BLOOD PRESSURE PERCENTILE*	SYSTOLIC BLOOD PRESSURE BY PERCENTILE OF HEIGHT, MM Hg†							DIASTOLIC BLOOD PRESSURE BY PERCENTILE OF HEIGHT, MM Hg†						
		5%	10%	25%	50%	75%	90%	95%	5%	10%	25%	50%	75%	90%	95%
1	90th	97	98	99	100	102	103	104	53	53	53	54	55	56	56
	95th	101	102	103	104	105	107	107	57	57	57	58	59	60	60
2	90th	99	99	100	102	103	104	105	57	57	58	58	59	60	61
	95th	102	103	104	105	107	108	109	61	61	62	62	63	64	65
3	90th	100	100	102	103	104	105	106	61	61	61	62	63	63	64
	95th	104	104	105	107	108	109	110	65	65	65	66	67	67	68
4	90th	101	102	103	104	106	107	108	63	63	64	65	65	66	67
	95th	105	106	107	108	109	111	111	67	67	68	69	69	70	71
5	90th	103	103	104	106	107	108	109	65	66	66	67	68	68	69
	95th	107	107	108	110	111	112	113	69	70	70	71	72	72	73
6	90th	104	105	106	107	109	110	111	67	67	68	69	69	70	71
	95th	108	109	110	111	112	114	114	71	71	72	73	73	74	75
7	90th	106	107	108	109	110	112	112	69	69	69	70	71	72	72
	95th	110	110	112	113	114	115	116	73	73	73	74	75	76	76
8	90th	108	109	110	111	112	113	114	70	70	71	71	72	73	74
	95th	112	112	113	115	116	117	118	74	74	75	75	76	77	78
9	90th	110	110	112	113	114	115	116	71	72	72	73	74	74	75

Age	Percentile														
10	95th	114	114	115	117	118	119	120	75	76	76	77	78	78	79
	90th	112	112	114	115	116	117	118	73	73	73	74	75	76	76
11	95th	116	116	117	119	120	121	122	77	77	77	78	79	80	80
	90th	114	114	116	117	118	119	120	74	74	75	75	76	77	77
12	95th	118	118	119	121	122	123	124	78	78	79	79	80	81	81
	90th	116	116	118	119	120	121	122	75	75	76	76	77	78	78
13	95th	120	120	121	123	124	125	126	79	79	80	80	81	82	82
	90th	118	118	119	121	122	123	124	76	76	77	78	78	79	80
14	95th	121	122	122	125	126	127	128	80	80	81	82	82	83	84
	90th	119	120	121	122	124	125	126	77	77	78	79	79	80	81
15	95th	123	124	125	126	128	129	130	81	81	82	83	83	84	85
	90th	121	121	122	124	125	126	127	78	78	79	79	80	81	82
16	95th	124	125	126	128	129	130	131	82	82	83	83	84	85	86
	90th	122	122	123	125	126	127	128	79	79	79	80	81	82	82
17	95th	125	126	127	128	130	131	132	83	83	83	84	85	86	86
	90th	122	123	124	125	126	128	128	79	79	79	80	81	82	82

From Update on Task force report on high blood pressure in children, 1996.
Blood pressure percentile was determined by a single reading.
†*Height percentile was determined by standard growth curves.*

CLINICAL AND
REFERENCE NOTES

CHAPTER 11

BREASTS AND AXILLAE

EQUIPMENT

- Ruler (if mass detected)
- Flashlight with transilluminator (if mass detected)
- Glass slide and cytologic fixative (for nipple discharge)
- Small pillow or folded towel

EXAMINATION

TECHNIQUE	FINDINGS

Females

With patient seated and arms hanging loosely, inspect both breasts

Inspect all quadrants and tail of Spence as shown in the figure. If necessary, lift breasts with fingertips to expose lower and lateral aspects.

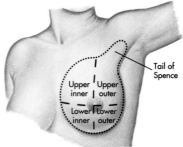

- *Size/shape/symmetry*

  EXPECTED: Convex, pendulous, or conical. Frequently asymmetric in size.

- *Texture/contour*

  EXPECTED: Smooth and uninterrupted.

  UNEXPECTED: Dimpling or peau d'orange appearance. Changes or asymmetric appearance.

TECHNIQUE	FINDINGS

- *Skin color*

EXPECTED: Consistent color.
UNEXPECTED: Areas of discoloration or asymmetric appearance.

- *Venous patterns*

EXPECTED: Bilateral venous networks, although pronounced generally only in pregnant or obese women.
UNEXPECTED: Unilateral network.

- *Markings*

EXPECTED: Long-standing nevi. Supernumerary nipples possible (but could be a clue to other congenital abnormalities).
UNEXPECTED: Changing or tender nevi. Lesions.

Inspect areolae and nipples

- *Size/shape/symmetry*

EXPECTED: Areolae round or oval, bilaterally equal or nearly equal. Nipples bilaterally equal or nearly equal in size and usually everted, although one or both sometimes inverted.
UNEXPECTED: Recent unilateral nipple inversion or retraction.

- *Color*

EXPECTED: Areolae and nipples pink to brown.
UNEXPECTED: Nonhomogeneous in color.

- *Texture/contour*

EXPECTED: Areolae smooth, except for Montgomery tubercles. Nipples smooth or wrinkled.

TECHNIQUE   FINDINGS

UNEXPECTED: Areolae with suppurative or tender Montgomery tubercles or with peau d'orange appearance. Nipples crusting, cracking, or with discharge.

With patient in the following positions, reinspect both breasts

- *Arms extended over head*

- *Hands pressed on hips or pushed together in front of chest*
- *Seated and leaning over*
- *Recumbent*

EXPECTED, ALL POSITIONS: Breasts bilaterally equal with even contour.
UNEXPECTED: Dimpling, retraction, deviation, or fixation of breasts.

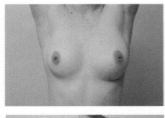 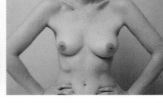

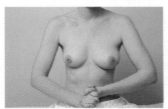 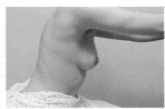

TECHNIQUE	FINDINGS

With patient seated and arms hanging loosely, palpate breasts

First palpate entire breast lightly, then repeat with deeper, heavier palpation. Using finger pads, systematically palpate both breasts in all four quadrants and over the areolae. Push gently but firmly toward chest while rotating fingers clockwise or counterclockwise, following a *vertical strip, concentric circle,* or *wedge* pattern. For large breasts, perform bimanual palpation, immobilizing inferior surface with one hand while examining superior surface with the other hand.

EXPECTED: Tissue generally dense, firm, and elastic, but sometimes lobular. The inframammary ridge may be felt along lower edge of breast. During menstrual cycle, cyclic pattern of breast enlargement, increased nodularity, and tenderness.

UNEXPECTED: Lumps or nodules. Characterize any masses by location, size, shape, consistency, tenderness, mobility, delineation of borders, and retraction. Use transillumination to assess presence of fluid in masses.

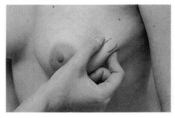

With patient seated and arms raised over her head, palpate tail of Spence

Gently compress tissue between thumb and fingers.

EXPECTED: Similar to expected findings above, with patient's arms hanging loosely.

UNEXPECTED: Similar to unexpected findings above with patient's arms hanging loosely.

TECHNIQUE	**FINDINGS**

With patient seated and arms flexed at the elbows, palpate for lymph nodes.

Left side. Support patient's lower right arm with your right hand while examining the left axilla with your left hand. With palmar surface of fingers, reach deep into hollow, pushing firmly upward, then bring fingers down, gently rolling soft tissue against chest wall and axilla. Explore apex, medial, and lateral aspects along rib cage; lateral aspects along upper surface of arm; and anterior and posterior walls of axilla. Hook fingers over clavicle and rotate over supraclavicular area while patient turns head toward same side and raises shoulder.
Repeat on left side.

UNEXPECTED: Nodes, especially in supraclavicular area. Describe nodes by location, size, shape, consistency, tenderness, fixation, and delineation of borders.

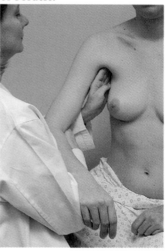

Palpate and compress nipples

Gently compress between thumb and index finger as shown.

EXPECTED: Possible nipple erection and areola puckering.
UNEXPECTED: Discharge. Note color and origin of any discharge and prepare smear.

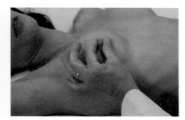

TECHNIQUE	FINDINGS

With patient supine, continue palpation of breast tissue

Have patient put one hand behind head. Place a towel under shoulder of same side. Compress breast tissue between fingers and chest wall, using rotary motion of fingers. Have patient place arm at her side, and repeat palpation. Repeat with other breast.

EXPECTED: Similar to expectations of patient seated, with arms hanging loosely.
UNEXPECTED: Similar to unexpected findings of patient seated, with arms hanging loosely.

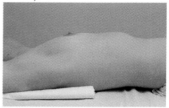

Males

Inspect both breasts
- *Size/shape/symmetry*
- *Surface characteristics*

EXPECTED: Even with chest wall. Sometimes convex (especially overweight men).
UNEXPECTED: Enlarged breasts.

Inspect areolae and nipples
- *Size/shape/symmetry*

EXPECTED: Areolae round or oval, bilaterally equal or nearly equal. Nipples bilaterally equal or nearly equal in size and usually everted, although one or both sometimes inverted.
UNEXPECTED: Recent unilateral nipple inversion or retraction.

- *Color*

EXPECTED: Areolae and nipples pink to brown.
UNEXPECTED: Nonhomogenous in color.

TECHNIQUE	FINDINGS

■ *Texture/contour*

EXPECTED: Areolae smooth, except for Montgomery tubercles. Nipples smooth or wrinkled.
UNEXPECTED: Areolae with suppurative or tender Montgomery tubercles or with peau d'orange appearance. Nipples crusting, cracking, or with discharge.

Palpate breasts and over areolae

Palpate briefly, following palpation steps for "females."

EXPECTED: Thin layer of fatty tissue overlying muscle. Thick layer in obese men may give appearance of breast enlargement. Firm disk of glandular tissue sometimes evident.
UNEXPECTED: Lumps or nodules.

With patient seated and arms flexed at the elbows, palpate for lymph nodes

Palpate as described for "females."

UNEXPECTED: Nodes, especially in supraclavicular area. Describe nodes by location, size, shape, consistency, tenderness, fixation, and delineation of borders.

Palpate and compress nipples

Gently compress between thumb and index finger.

EXPECTED: Possible nipple erection and areola puckering.
UNEXPECTED: Discharge. Note color and origin of any discharge and prepare smear.

AIDS TO DIFFERENTIAL DIAGNOSIS

ABNORMALITY	DESCRIPTION
Fibrocystic disease	See table of differentiating signs
Fibroadenoma	and symptoms on p. 143.
Malignant breast tumors	
Adult gynecomastia	Smooth, firm, mobile, tender disk of breast tissue behind areola in males, unilaterally or bilaterally.
Mastitis	Swelling, tenderness, heat; patient may have fever. Abscess—pus-filled hardened mass that is fluctuant, hard, and erythematous.

PEDIATRIC VARIATIONS

EXAMINATION

TECHNIQUE	FINDINGS
Palpate and compress nipples	
	EXPECTED: Breast enlargement is not unusual in newborns. "Witch's milk" may be expressed.

AIDS TO DIFFERENTIAL DIAGNOSIS

ABNORMALITY	DESCRIPTION
Gynecomastia	Enlargement of breast tissue in boys caused by puberty, hormonal unbalance, testicular or pituitary tumors, or medications containing estrogens or steroids. Thorough investigation should be conducted to rule out pathologic conditions.

Differentiating Signs and Symptoms of Breast Masses

	FIBROCYSTIC DISEASE	FIBROADENOMA	CANCER
Age	20-49	15-55	30-80
Occurrence	Usually bilateral	Usually bilateral	Usually unilateral
Number	Multiple or single	Single; may be multiple	Single
Shape	Round	Round or discoid	Irregular or stellate
Consistency	Soft to firm; tense	Firm, rubbery	Hard, stonelike
Mobility	Mobile	Mobile	Fixed
Retraction signs	Absent	Absent	Often present
Tenderness	Usually tender	Usually nontender	Usually nontender
Delimitation	Well delineated	Well delineated	Poorly delineated; irregular
Variation with menses	Yes	No	No

Females

Breasts. Moderate size, conical shape, left slightly larger than right. No skin lesions, contour smooth without dimpling or retraction; venous pattern symmetrical. Nipple symmetric without discharge; Montgomery tubercles bilaterally. Tissue dense, particularly in upper quadrants. No palpable masses. No supraclavicular, infraclavicular, or axillary lymphadenopathy.

Males

Breasts. Small, bilaterally symmetric with male contour. No skin or nipple lesions; no nipple discharge. Tissue smooth without palpable masses. No palpable supraclavicular, infraclavicular, or axillary lymph nodes.

CHAPTER 12

ABDOMEN

EQUIPMENT

- Stethoscope
- Marking pen
- Centimeter ruler or measuring tape
- Reflex hammer or tongue blade

EXAMINATION

Have patient in the supine position to start the examination.

TECHNIQUE	FINDINGS

Inspect abdomen in all four quadrants (see the box on p. 146)

- *Skin color/characteristics*

EXPECTED: Usual color variations, such as paleness or tanning lines. Fine venous network (venous return toward head above umbilicus, toward feet below umbilicus).

UNEXPECTED: Generalized color changes, such as jaundice or cyanosis. Glistening taut appearance. Bluish periumbilical discoloration, bruises, and other localized discoloration. Striae, lesions or nodules, a pearl-like enlarged umbilical node, and scars.

Anatomic Correlates of the Four Quadrants of the Abdomen

RIGHT UPPER QUADRANT	*LEFT UPPER QUADRANT*
Liver and gallbladder	Left lobe of liver
Pylorus	Spleen
Duodenum	Stomach
Head of pancreas	Body of pancreas
Right adrenal gland	Left adrenal gland
Portion of right kidney	Portion of left kidney
Hepatic flexure of colon	Splenic flexure of colon
Portions of ascending and transverse colon	Portions of transverse and descending colon
RIGHT LOWER QUADRANT	*LEFT LOWER QUADRANT*
Lower pole of right kidney	Lower pole of left kidney
Cecum and appendix	Sigmoid colon
Portion of ascending colon	Portion of descending colon
Bladder (if distended)	Bladder (if distended)
Ovary and salpinx	Ovary and salpinx
Uterus (if enlarged)	Uterus (if enlarged)
Right spermatic cord	Left spermatic cord
Right ureter	Left ureter

From Thompson and Wilson, 1996.

TECHNIQUE

- *Contour/symmetry*
  Begin seated to patient's right to enhance shadows and contouring. Inspect while patient breathes comfortably and while patient holds a deep breath. Assess symmetry, first seated at patient's side, then standing behind patient's head.

FINDINGS

EXPECTED: Flat, rounded, or scaphoid. Contralateral areas symmetric. Maximum height of convexity at umbilicus. Abdomen remains smooth and symmetric while holding breath.

UNEXPECTED: Umbilicus displaced upward, downward, or laterally, or inflamed, swollen, or bulging. Any distention (symmetric or asymmetric), bulges, or masses while breathing comfortably or holding breath.

TECHNIQUE	FINDINGS
■ *Surface motion*	**EXPECTED:** Smooth, even motion with respiration, females mostly costal, males mostly abdominal. Pulsation in upper midline in thin adults. **UNEXPECTED:** Limited motion with respiration in adult males. Rippling movement (peristalsis) or marked pulsation.

Inspect abdominal muscles as patient raises head

	EXPECTED: No masses or protrusions. **UNEXPECTED:** Masses, protrusion of the umbilicus and other hernia signs, or muscle separation.

Auscultate with stethoscope diaphragm

■ *Frequency and character of bowel sounds* Warm stethoscope diaphragm and hold with light pressure. Auscultate in all quadrants.	**EXPECTED:** 5 to 35 irregular clicks and gurgles per minute. Borborygmi or increased sounds due to hunger. **UNEXPECTED:** Increased sounds unrelated to hunger, high-pitched tinkling, or decreased or absent sounds.
■ *Liver and spleen*	**EXPECTED:** Silent. **UNEXPECTED:** Friction rubs.

Auscultate with stethoscope bell

■ *Vascular sounds* Listen with stethoscope bell in all quadrants.	**EXPECTED:** No bruits, venous hum, or friction rubs. **UNEXPECTED:** Bruits in aortic, renal, iliac, or femoral arteries.
■ *Epigastric region and around umbilicus*	**EXPECTED:** No venous hum. **UNEXPECTED:** Venous hum.

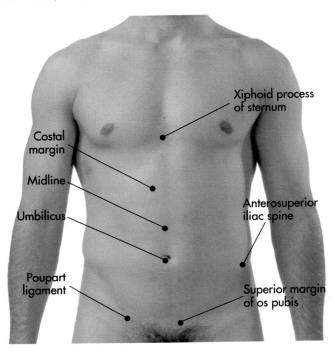

Percussion Notes of the Abdomen		
NOTE	**DESCRIPTION**	**LOCATION**
Tympany	Musical note of higher pitch than resonance	Over air-filled viscera
Hyperresonance	Pitch lies between tympany and resonance	Base of left lung
Resonance	Sustained note of moderate pitch	Over lung tissue and sometimes over the abdomen
Dullness	Short, high-pitched note with little resonance	Over solid organs adjacent to air-filled structures

Modified from AH Robins Co.

TECHNIQUE	FINDINGS

Percuss abdomen

  NOTE: Percussion can be done independently or concurrently with palpation.

- *Tone*
  Percuss in all quadrants.

  EXPECTED: Tympany predominant. Dullness over organs and solid masses. Dullness in suprapubic area from distended bladder. See the table on p. 148 for percussion notes.
  UNEXPECTED: Dullness predominant.

- *Liver span*
  Upper edge of liver is detected by percussing at right midclavicular line over area of tympany. To determine lower liver border, percuss upward as shown in the figure at right and mark with pen where tympany changes to dullness. To determine upper liver border, percuss downward as shown and mark change to dullness. Measure the distance between marks to estimate vertical span.

  EXPECTED: Lower border usually begins at or slightly below costal margin. Upper border usually begins at fifth to seventh intercostal space. Span generally ranges from 6 to 12 cm in adults.
  UNEXPECTED: Lower liver border more than 2 to 3 cm below costal margin. Upper liver border below seventh or above fifth intercostal span. Span greater than 12 cm or less than 6 cm.

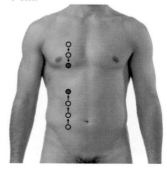

From Thompson and Wilson, 1996.

TECHNIQUE	FINDINGS

- *Spleen*
Percuss just posterior to midaxillary line on left, beginning at areas of lung resonance and moving in several directions. Percuss lowest intercostal space in left anterior axillary line before and after patient takes deep breath.

EXPECTED: Small area of dullness from sixth to tenth rib. Tympany before and after deep breath.
UNEXPECTED: Large area of dullness (check for full stomach or feces-filled intestine). Tone change from tympany to dullness with inspiration.

- *Stomach*
Percuss in area of left lower anterior rib cage and left epigastric region.

EXPECTED: Tympany of gastric air bubble (lower than intestine tympany).
UNEXPECTED: Dullness.

Lightly palpate abdomen

Stand at patient's side (usually right). Systematically palpate all quadrants, avoiding areas previously identified as trouble spots. With palmar surfaces of fingers, depress abdominal wall up to 1 cm with light, even motion.
Identify areas of peritoneal irritation by assessing for cutaneous hypersensitivity.

EXPECTED: Abdomen smooth with consistent softness. Possible tension from palpating too deeply, cold hands, or ticklishness.
UNEXPECTED: Muscular tension or resistance, tenderness, or masses. If resistance is present, place pillow under patient's knees, and ask patient to breathe slowly through mouth. Feel for relaxation of rectus abdominis muscles on expiration. Continuing tension signals involuntary response to abdominal rigidity. Cutaneous hypersensitivity.

Palpate abdomen with moderate pressure

Using same hand position as above, palpate all quadrants again, this time with moderate pressure.

EXPECTED: Soft, nontender.
UNEXPECTED: Tenderness.

TECHNIQUE	FINDINGS

Deeply palpate abdomen

With same hand position as above, repeat palpation in all quadrants, pressing deeply and evenly into abdominal wall. Move fingers back and forth over abdominal contents. Use bimanual technique—exerting pressure with top hand and concentrating on sensation with bottom hand, as shown in the figure at right—if obesity or muscular resistance makes deep palpation difficult. To help determine if masses are superficial or intraabdominal, have patient lift head from examining table to contract abdominal muscles and obscure intraabdominal masses.

EXPECTED: Possible sensation of abdominal wall sliding back and forth. Possible awareness of borders of rectus abdominis muscles, aorta, and portions of colon. Possible tenderness over cecum, sigmoid colon, aorta, and in midline near xiphoid process.

UNEXPECTED: Bulges, masses, and tenderness, unrelated to deep palpation of cecum, sigmoid colon, aorta, and xiphoid process. Note location, size, shape, consistency, tenderness, pulsation, mobility, and movement (with respiration) of any masses.

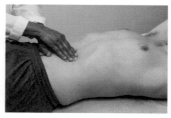

■ *Umbilical ring and umbilicus*

Palpate umbilical ring and around umbilicus. Note whether ring is incomplete or soft in center.

EXPECTED: Umbilical ring circular and free of irregularities. Umbilicus either slightly inverted or everted.

UNEXPECTED: Bulges, nodules, and granulation. Protruding umbilicus.

TECHNIQUE	FINDINGS

- *Liver*
  Place left hand under patient at eleventh and twelfth ribs, lifting to elevate liver toward abdominal wall. Place right hand on abdomen, fingers extended toward head with tips on right midclavicular line below level of liver dullness, as shown in the figure at right. Alternately, place right hand parallel to right costal margin, as shown in the figure at right, below. Press right hand gently but deeply in and up. Ask patient to breathe comfortably a few times and then take a deep breath. Feel for liver edge as diaphragm pushes it down. If palpable repeat maneuver medially and laterally to costal margin.

EXPECTED: Usually liver is not palpable. If felt, liver edge should be firm, smooth, and even.

UNEXPECTED: Tenderness, nodules, or irregularity.

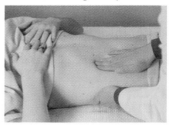

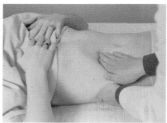

- *Gallbladder*
  Palpate below liver margin at lateral border of rectus abdominis muscle.

EXPECTED: Gallbladder not palpable.

UNEXPECTED: Palpable, tender or nontender. If tender (possible cholecystitis), palpate deeply during inspiration and observe for pain (Murphy sign).

TECHNIQUE   **FINDINGS**

■ *Spleen*

Reach across patient with left hand, place it beneath patient over left costovertebral angle, and lift spleen anteriorly toward abdominal wall. As shown in the figure, place right hand on abdomen below left costal margin and—using findings from percussion—gently press fingertips inward toward spleen while asking patient to take a deep breath. Feel for spleen as it moves downward toward fingers. Repeat with patient lying on right side, as shown in the figure below, with hips and knees flexed. Press inward with left hand while using fingertips of right hand to feel edge of spleen.

EXPECTED: Spleen usually not palpable by either method.
UNEXPECTED: Palpable spleen.

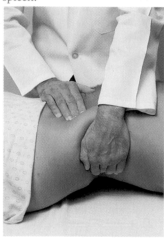

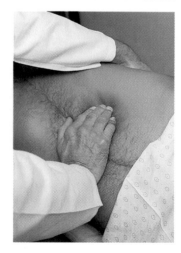

TECHNIQUE	FINDINGS

- *Left kidney*
Standing on patient's right, reach across with left hand and place over left flank, then place right hand at patient's left costal margin. Ask patient to inhale deeply, while you elevate left flank and palpate deeply with right hand.

EXPECTED: Left kidney usually not palpable.
UNEXPECTED: Pain.

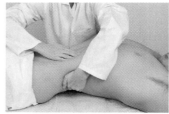

- *Right kidney*
Standing on patient's right, place left hand under right flank, then place right hand at patient's right costal margin. Ask patient to inhale deeply while you elevate right flank and palpate deeply with right hand.

EXPECTED: If palpable, right kidney should be smooth and firm with rounded edges.
UNEXPECTED: Tenderness.

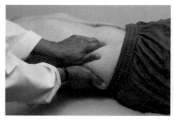

- *Aorta*
Palpate deeply slightly to left of midline, and feel for aortic pulsation. As an alternate technique, place palmar surface of hands with fingers extended on midline and press fingers deeply inward on each side of aorta and feel for pulsation. For thin patients, use one hand, placing thumb and fingers on either side of aorta.

EXPECTED: Pulsation anterior in direction.
UNEXPECTED: Prominent lateral pulsation.

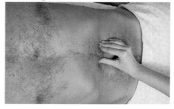

TECHNIQUE	FINDINGS

■ *Urinary bladder*
Percuss distended bladder to help determine outline, then palpate.

EXPECTED: Ordinarily not palpable unless distended with urine. If distended, bladder should be smooth, round, and tense, and on percussion will elicit lower note than surrounding air-filled intestines.
UNEXPECTED: Palpable when not distended with urine.

Elicit abdominal reflexes

Stroke each quadrant of abdomen with end of reflex hammer or tongue blade edge. Elicit upper abdominal reflexes by stroking upward and away from umbilicus; elicit lower abdominal reflexes by stroking downward and away from umbilicus.

EXPECTED: With each stroke, contraction of rectus abdominis muscles and pulling of umbilicus toward stroked side. Reflex may be diminished in patient who is obese or whose abdominal muscles were stretched during pregnancy.
UNEXPECTED: Absence of reflex.

With patient sitting, percuss costovertebral angles

Stand behind patient. Right side: Place left hand over right costovertebral angle and strike hand with ulnar surface of left fist. Left side: Repeat with hands reversed.

EXPECTED: No tenderness.
UNEXPECTED: Kidney tenderness or pain.

Pain assessment

Keep eyes on patient's face while examining abdomen. To help characterize pain, have patient cough, take a deep breath, jump, or walk. Ask if patient is hungry.

UNEXPECTED: Unwillingness to move, nausea, vomiting, and areas of localized tenderness. Lack of hunger. See the box on p. 156 and the table on p. 158.

Some Causes of Pain Perceived in Anatomic Regions

RIGHT UPPER QUADRANT
Duodenal ulcer
Hepatitis
Hepatomegaly
Pneumonia

LEFT UPPER QUADRANT
Ruptured spleen
Gastric ulcer
Aortic aneurysm
Perforated colon
Pneumonia

RIGHT LOWER QUADRANT
Appendicitis
Salpingitis
Ovarian cyst
Ruptured ectopic pregnancy
Renal/ureteral stone
Strangulated hernia
Meckel diverticulitis
Regional ileitis
Perforated cecum

LEFT LOWER QUADRANT
Sigmoid diverticulitis
Salpingitis
Ovarian cyst
Ruptured ectopic pregnancy
Renal/ureteral stone
Strangulated hernia
Perforated colon
Regional ileitis
Ulcerative colitis

PERIUMBILICAL
Intestinal obstruction
Acute pancreatitis
Early appendicitis
Mesenteric thrombosis
Aortic aneurysm
Diverticulitis

Modified from Judge et al, 1988.

TECHNIQUE	FINDINGS

Iliopsoas muscle test

Use test for suspected appendicitis. With patient supine, place hand over lower thigh. Ask patient to raise leg, flexing at hip, while you push downward.

UNEXPECTED: Lower quadrant pain.

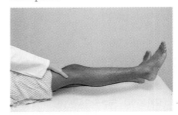

TECHNIQUE	FINDINGS

Obturator muscle test

Use test for suspected ruptured appendix or pelvic abscess. With patient supine, ask patient to flex right leg at hip and bend knee to 90 degrees. Hold leg just above knee, grasp ankle, and rotate leg laterally and medially, as shown in the figure at right.

UNEXPECTED: Pain in hypogastric region.

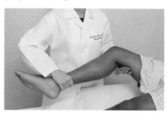

AIDS TO DIFFERENTIAL DIAGNOSIS

ABNORMALITY	DESCRIPTION
Hiatal hernia with esophagitis	Epigastric pain and/or heartburn that worsens with reclining and is relieved by sitting or with antacids; water brash; or dysphagia. Sudden onset of vomiting, pain, and complete dysphagia are symptoms of hernia incarceration.
Duodenal ulcer	Localized epigastric pain occurring with empty stomach that is relieved with food or antacids. Tenderness on palpation of abdomen for anterior-wall ulcers. Hematemesis, melena, dizziness or syncope, decreased blood pressure, increased pulse rate, and decreased hematocrit level are symptoms of upper gastrointestinal (GI) bleeding. Signs of an acute abdomen could indicate perforation of duodenum, **a life-threatening event.**

Abdominal Signs Associated With Common Abnormalities

SIGN	DESCRIPTION
Aaron	Pain or distress occurs in the area of the patient's heart or stomach on palpation of McBurney point
Ballance	Fixed dullness to percussion in left flank, and dullness in right flank that disappears on change of position
Blumberg	Rebound tenderness
Cullen	Ecchymosis around umbilicus
Dance	Absence of bowel sounds in right lower quadrant
Grey Turner	Ecchymosis of flanks
Kehr	Abdominal pain radiating to left shoulder
Markle (heel jar)	Patient stands with straightened knees, then raises up on toes, relaxes, and allows heels to hit floor, thus jarring body. Action will cause abdominal pain if positive
McBurney	Rebound tenderness and sharp pain when McBurney point is palpated
Murphy	Abrupt cessation of inspiration on palpation of gallbladder
Romberg-Howship	Pain down the medial aspect of the thigh to the knees
Rovsing	Right lower quadrant pain intensified by left lower quadrant abdominal palpation

ASSOCIATED CONDITIONS

Appendicitis

Peritoneal irritation

Peritoneal irritation; appendicitis

Hemoperitoneum; pancreatitis; ectopic pregnancy

Intussusception

Hemoperitoneum; pancreatitis

Spleen rupture; renal calculi; ectopic pregnancy

Peritoneal irritation; appendicitis

Appendicitis

Cholecystitis

Strangulated obturator hernia

Peritoneal irritation; appendicitis

ABNORMALITY	DESCRIPTION
Crohn disease	Cramping diarrhea, mild bleeding, occurs anywhere in GI tract; fissure, fistula abscess formation; periumbilical colic; malabsorption; folate deficiency.
Ulcerative colitis	Mild to severe symptoms; bloody, watery diarrhea; no localized peritoneal signs; weight loss, fatigue, general debility.
Colon cancer	Occult blood in stool. History of changes in frequency or character of stool. Lesion felt on rectal examination. Tumor palpated in right or left lower quadrant.
Hepatitis	Jaundice, anorexia, abdominal gastric discomfort, clay-colored stools, tea-colored urine. Enlarged liver. Caused by viral infection, alcohol, drugs, or toxins.
Cirrhosis	Ascites, jaundice, prominent abdominal vasculature, cutaneous spider angiomas, dark urine, light-colored stools, and spleen enlargement. Complaints of fatigue. Muscle wasting in late stages.
Cholecystitis	*Acute:* Pain in upper right quadrant with radiation around midtorso to right scapular region. Pain abrupt and severe, lasting 2 to 4 hours. *Chronic:* Repeated acute attacks; a scarred and contracted gallbladder; fat intolerance, flatulence, nausea, anorexia, and nonspecific abdominal pain and tenderness of right hypochondriac region.

Differential Diagnosis of Urinary Incontinence

CONDITION	HISTORY	PHYSICAL FINDINGS
Stress incontinence	Small-volume incontinence with cough, sneezing, laughing, running; history of prior pelvic surgery	Pelvic floor relaxation; cystocele, rectocele; lax urethral sphincter; loss of urine with provoacative testing; atrophic vaginitis; postvoid residual <100 ml
Urge incontinence	Uncontrolled urge to void; large-volume incontinence; history of central nervous system (CNS) disorders such as stroke, multiple sclerosis, parkinsonism	Unexpected findings only as related to CNS disorder; postvoid residual <100 ml
Overflow incontinence	Small-volume incontinence, dribbling; hesitancy; In men symptoms of enlarged prostate—nocturia, dribbling, hesitancy, deceased force and caliber of stream	Distended bladder; prostate hypertrophy; stool in rectum, fecal impaction; postvoid residual >100 ml
	In neurogenic bladder: history of bowel problems, spinal cord injury, or multiple sclerosis	Evidence of spinal cord disease or diabetic neuropathy; lax sphincter; gait disturbance
Functional incontinence	Change in mental status, impaired mobility, new environment	Impaired mental status; impaired mobility
	Medications: hypnotics, diuretics, anticholinergic agents, alpha-adrenergic agents, calcium channel blockers	Impaired mental status or unexpected findings only as related to other physical conditions

ABNORMALITY	DESCRIPTION
Chronic pancreatitis	Unremitting abdominal pain, epigastric tenderness, weight loss, steatorrhea, and glucose intolerance.
Pyelonephritis	Flank pain, bacteriuria, pyuria, dysuria, nocturia, and urinary frequency. Possible costovertebral angle tenderness.
Renal calculi	Fever, hematuria, and flank pain that may extend to groin and genitals.
Appendicitis	Initially, periumbilical or epigastric pain; colicky; later becomes localized to right lower quadrant, often at McBurney point.

PEDIATRIC VARIATIONS

EXAMINATION

TECHNIQUE	FINDINGS

Inspect abdomen in all four quadrants

The infant's abdomen should be examined, if possible, during a time of relaxation and quiet. Sucking on a bottle or pacifier may help to relax the infant.

- *Contour/symmetry* — **EXPECTED:** In children, the abdomen will be protuberant until age 3 when standing.

- *Surface motion* — **EXPECTED:** Pulsation in epigastric area in infants.
  UNEXPECTED: Peristaltic waves associated with pyloric stenosis.

TECHNIQUE	FINDINGS
Percuss abdomen	
■ *Tone*	**EXPECTED:** More tympany is present in children than adults.
Deeply palpate abdomen	
■ *Umbilical ring*	**EXPECTED:** Children up to 4 years old may have an umbilical hernia.
■ *Liver*	**EXPECTED:** Liver may be palpable in young children 2 to 3 cm below the costal margin.

AGE	LIVER SPAN (CM)
6 months	2.4-2.8
12 months	2.8-3.1
24 months	3.5-3.6
3 years	4.0
4 years	4.3-4.4
5 years	4.5-5.1
6 years	4.8-5.1
8 years	5.1-5.6
10 years	5.5-6.1

SAMPLE DOCUMENTATION

Abdomen. Rounded and symmetric with white striae adjacent to umbilicus in all quadrants. A well healed 5-cm white surgical scar evident in right lower quadrant. No areas of visible pulsations or peristalsis. Active bowel sounds audible all four quadrants. Percussion tones tympanic over epigastrium and resonant over remainder of abdomen. Liver span 8 cm at right midclavicular line (MCL). On inspiration, liver edge firm, smooth, and nontender. No splenomegaly. Musculature soft and relaxed to light palpation. No masses or areas of tenderness to deep palpation. Superficial reflexes intact. No costovertebral angle tenderness.

CLINICAL AND
REFERENCE NOTES

CHAPTER 13

FEMALE GENITALIA

EQUIPMENT

- Gloves
- Sterile cotton swabs
- Culture plates
- Cytologic fixative
- Speculum
- Water-soluble lubricant
- Lamp
- Wooden or plastic spatula
- Glass slides
- Cervical brushes
- DNA probe kits for *Chlamydia*/gonorrhea

EXAMINATION

Have patient in lithotomy position, draped for minimal exposure.

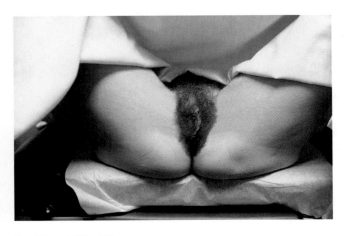

From Edge and Miller, 1994.

TECHNIQUE   FINDINGS

External Genitalia

Wear gloves on both hands

Ask patient to separate or drop open her knees. Tell patient you are beginning examination, then touch either lower thigh and—without breaking contact—move hand along thigh to external genitalia.

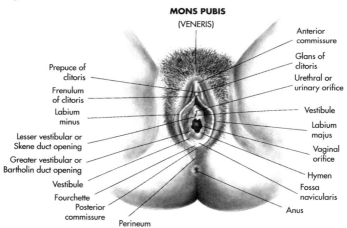

Inspect and palpate mons pubis

- *Characteristics*

  EXPECTED: Skin smooth and clean.
  UNEXPECTED: Improper hygiene.

- *Pubic hair*

  EXPECTED: Regularly distributed female pubic hair.
  UNEXPECTED: Nits or lice.

Inspect and palpate labia

- *Labia majora*

  EXPECTED: Gaping or closed, dry or moist, shriveled or full, tissue soft and homogeneous, usually symmetric.

TECHNIQUE	FINDINGS

UNEXPECTED: Swelling, redness, tenderness, discoloration, varicosities, obvious stretching, or signs of trauma or scarring. If excoriation, rashes, or lesions are present, ask patient if she has been scratching.

■ *Labia minora*
Separate labia majora with fingers of one hand. With other hand, palpate labia minora between thumb and second finger.

EXPECTED: Moist, dark-pink inner surface. Tissue soft and homogeneous.
UNEXPECTED: Tenderness, inflammation, irritation, excoriation, caking of discharge in tissue folds, discoloration, ulcers, vesicles, irregularities, or nodules. Hyperemia of fourchette not related to recent sexual activity.

Inspect clitoris
■ *Size and length*

EXPECTED: Length 2 cm or less; diameter 0.5 cm
UNEXPECTED: Enlargement, atrophy, inflammation, or adhesions.

Inspect urethral meatus and vaginal opening
■ *Urethral orifice*

EXPECTED: Slit or irregular opening, close to or in vaginal introitus, and usually midline.
UNEXPECTED: Discharge, polyps, caruncles, fistulas, lesions, irritation, inflammation, or dilation.

■ *Vaginal introitus*

EXPECTED: Thin vertical slit or large orifice with irregular edges. Tissue moist.

TECHNIQUE	FINDINGS

UNEXPECTED: Swelling, discoloration, discharge, lesions, fistulas, or fissures.

Milk Skene glands

Tell patient you will be inserting one finger in her vagina and pressing forward with it. With palm up, insert index finger to second joint, press upward, and milk Skene glands by moving finger outward. Perform on both sides of urethra and directly on urethra.

UNEXPECTED: Discharge or tenderness. Note color, consistency, and odor of any discharge; obtain culture.

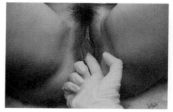

Palpate Bartholin glands

Tell patient she will feel you pressing around entrance to vagina. Palpate lateral tissue between index finger and thumb, then palpate entire area bilaterally, particularly posterolateral portion of labia majora.

EXPECTED: No swelling.
UNEXPECTED: Swelling, tenderness, masses, heat, fluctuation, or discharge. Note color, consistency, and odor of any discharge; obtain culture.

Test vaginal muscle tone

Ask patient to squeeze vaginal opening around your finger.

EXPECTED: Fairly tight squeezing by some nulliparous women, less so by some multiparous women.
UNEXPECTED: Protrusion of cervix or uterus.

Inspect for bulging and urinary incontinence

Ask patient to bear down.

EXPECTED: No bulging.

TECHNIQUE	FINDINGS

UNEXPECTED: Bulging of anterior or posterior wall, or urinary incontinence.

Inspect and palpate perineum

Compress perineum tissue between finger and thumb

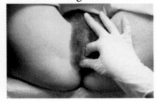

From Edge and Miller, 1994.

EXPECTED: Perineum surface smooth—generally thick and smooth in a nulliparous woman, thinner and rigid in a multiparous woman. Possible episiotomy scarring in women who have borne children.

UNEXPECTED: Tenderness, inflammation, fistulas, lesions, or growths.

Inspect anus

■ *Skin characteristics*

EXPECTED: Skin darkly pigmented and possibly coarse.

UNEXPECTED: Scarring, lesions, inflammation, fissures, lumps, skin tags, or excoriation.

Internal Genitalia—Speculum Examination

If you touched the perineum or anal skin while examining the external genitalia, change gloves before beginning internal examination.

Lubricate speculum and gloved fingers with water (if you expect to take specimens for analysis) or water-soluble lubricant (if you do not).

TECHNIQUE   **FINDINGS**

Insert speculum

Tell patient she will feel
you touching her again,
then insert two fingers of
the hand not holding the
speculum just inside vaginal introitus and press
downward. Ask the patient
to breathe slowly and try
to consciously relax her
muscles. Use the fingers of
that hand to separate the
labia minora very widely
so that the hymenal open-
ing becomes clearly visi-
ble. Then slowly insert the
speculum along the path
of least resistance, often
slightly downward, avoid-
ing trauma to the urethra
and vaginal walls. Some
clinicians insert the speculum blades at an oblique
angle, others prefer to
keep the blades horizontal.
In either case avoid touching the clitoris, catching
pubic hair, or pinching
labial skin. Insert the
speculum the length of the
vaginal canal. Maintaining
downward pressure, open
speculum by pressing on
thumb piece. Sweep
speculum slowly upward
until cervix comes into
view. Adjust light, then
manipulate speculum far-
ther into vagina so that
cervix is well exposed

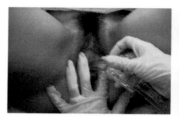

From Edge and Miller, 1994.

TECHNIQUE	FINDINGS

between anterior and posterior blades. Stabilize distal spread of blades and adjust proximal spread as needed.

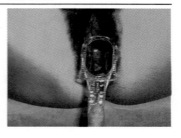

From Edge and Miller, 1994.

Inspect cervix

■ *Color*

EXPECTED: Evenly distributed pink. Symmetric, circumscribed erythema around os can be expected.
UNEXPECTED: Bluish, pale, or reddened cervix (especially if patchy or with irregular borders).

■ *Position*

EXPECTED: In midline, horizontal or pointing anteriorly or posteriorly. Protruding into vagina 1 to 3 cm.
UNEXPECTED: Deviation to right or left. Protrusion into vagina greater than 1 to 3 cm.

■ *Size*

EXPECTED: 3 cm in diameter.
UNEXPECTED: Larger than 3 cm.

■ *Shape*

EXPECTED: Uniform.
UNEXPECTED: Distorted.

■ *Surface characteristics*

EXPECTED: Surface smooth. Possible symmetric, reddened circle around os (squamocolumnar epithelium). Possible small, white, or yellow, raised round areas on cervix (nabothian cysts).

TECHNIQUE	FINDINGS

UNEXPECTED: Friable tissue, red patchy areas, granular areas, or white patches.

■ *Discharge*
Note any discharge. Determine origin: cervix or vagina.

EXPECTED: Odorless, creamy or clear, thick, thin, or stringy (often heavier at midcycle or immediately before menstruation).

UNEXPECTED: Odorous and white to yellow, green, or gray.

■ *Size and shape of os*

EXPECTED: Nulliparous woman: small, round, oval. Multiparous woman: usually a horizontal slit or irregular and stellate.

UNEXPECTED: Slit resulting from trauma from induced abortion, difficult removal of intrauterine device (IUD), or sexual abuse.

Collect vaginal smears and cultures

Follow standard precautions for safe collection of human secretions.

■ *Pap smear*
Collect sample from ectocervix with spatula. Insert longer projection of spatula into cervical os, rotate 360 degrees while keeping it flush against cervical tissue, then withdraw. Spread specimen on glass slide, spray with cytologic fixative, and label.

TECHNIQUE   **FINDINGS**

Insert brush device into cervical os until only bristles closest to handle are exposed, rotate $^1/_2$ to 1 turn, then withdraw. Roll and twist brush across glass slide, spray with cytologic fixative, and label. Warn patient that blood spotting might occur. (Vary technique appropriately for different types of brushes.)

- *Gonococcal culture specimen*

Insert sterile cotton swab into cervical os, hold in place for 10 to 30 seconds, then withdraw. Rotating swab, spread specimen in large Z pattern over culture medium and label. Follow agency routine for warming and transporting specimen.

If indicated, obtain anal culture: Insert fresh sterile cotton swab about 2.5 cm into rectum, rotate 360 degrees, hold for 10 to 30 seconds, and withdraw. Rotating swab, spread specimen in large Z pattern over culture medium and label.

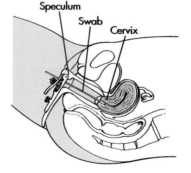

TECHNIQUE	FINDINGS

■ *DNA probe for* Chlamydia/*gonorrhea*
Remove excess mucus from ectocervix with swab and discard. Insert swab specified or provided by kit into cervical os and rotate for 30 seconds, then withdraw (avoiding vaginal walls). Place in transport tube, with swab in contact with reagent, and label. Follow agency procedure for testing, storage, and shipping.

■ *Wet mount and potassium hydroxide (KOH)*
Obtain a specimen of vaginal discharge using a swab. Smear the sample on a glass slide and add a drop of normal saline. Place a coverslip on the slide, and view under the microscope.

UNEXPECTED: The presence of trichomonads indicates *Trichomonas vaginalis.*
The presence of bacteria-filled epithelial cells (clue cells) indicates bacterial vaginosis.

On a separate glass slide place a specimen of vaginal discharge, apply a drop of aqueous 10% KOH, and put a coverslip in place.

UNEXPECTED: The presence of fishy odor (the "whiff test") suggests bacterial vaginosis.
View under the microscope for presence of mycelial fragments, hyphae, and budding yeast cells, which indicates candidiasis.

Withdraw speculum and inspect vaginal walls

Unlock speculum and remove it slowly, rotating it so vaginal walls can be inspected.
Maintain downward pressure and hook index finger

EXPECTED: Vaginal wall color same pink as cervix or lighter; moist, smooth or rugated; and homogeneous. Thin, clear or cloudy; odorless secretions.

TECHNIQUE	FINDINGS

over anterior blade as it is removed. Note odor of any discharge pooled in posterior blade, and obtain specimen if not already obtained.

UNEXPECTED: Reddened patches, lesions, pallor, cracks, bleeding, nodules, and swelling. Secretions that are profuse; thick, curdy, or frothy; gray, green, or yellow; or malodorous.

Internal Genitalia—Bimanual Examination

Change gloves, and then lubricate index and middle fingers of examining hand.

Tell patient you are going to examine her internally with your fingers. *Prevent thumb from touching clitoris during examination.*

Palpate vaginal wall while inserting fingers into vagina

Insert tips of index and middle fingers into vaginal opening and press downward, waiting for muscles to relax. Gradually insert fingers full length while palpating vaginal wall.

EXPECTED: Smooth and homogeneous.
UNEXPECTED: Tenderness, lesions, cysts, nodules, masses, or growths.

Palpate cervix

Locate cervix with palmar surface of fingers, feel end, and run fingers around circumference to feel fornices.

■ *Size, shape, and length*

EXPECTED: Consistent with speculum examination.

■ *Consistency*

EXPECTED: Firm in nonpregnant woman; softer in pregnant woman.
UNEXPECTED: Nodules, hardness, or roughness.

■ *Position*

EXPECTED: In midline horizontal or pointing anteriorly or posteriorly. Protruding into vagina 1 to 3 cm.

TECHNIQUE   **FINDINGS**

UNEXPECTED: Deviation to right or left. Protrusion into vagina greater than 1 to 3 cm.

■ *Mobility*
Grasp cervix gently between fingers and move from side to side. Observe patient's facial expression.

EXPECTED: 1 to 2 cm movement in each direction. Minimal discomfort.
UNEXPECTED: Pain on movement ("cervical motion tenderness").

Palpate uterus

■ *Location and position*
Place palmar surface of outside hand on abdominal midline, halfway between umbilicus and symphysis pubis, and place intravaginal fingers in anterior fornix. As shown in the figure at right, slowly slide outside hand toward pubis while pressing down and forward with flat surface of fingers; at the same time, push inward and up with fingertips of intravaginal hand while pushing down on cervix with backs of fingers. If uterus is anteverted or anteflexed, you should feel fundus between fingers of two hands at level of pubis.

If uterus cannot be felt with this maneuver, place intravaginal fingers together in posterior fornix and outside hand immediately above symphysis pu-

EXPECTED: In midline, horizontal, or pointing anteriorly or posteriorly. Protruding into vagina 1 to 3 cm.
UNEXPECTED: Deviation to right or left. Protrusion into vagina greater than 1 to 3 cm.

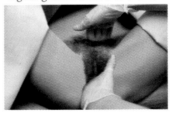

From Edge and Miller, 1994.

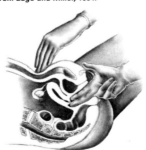

Anteverted

TECHNIQUE	FINDINGS

bis. Press firmly down with outside hand while pressing inward against cervix with intravaginal hand. If uterus is retroverted or retroflexed, you should feel fundus. If uterus cannot be felt with either of these maneuvers, move intravaginal fingers to each side of cervix and, while keeping contact with cervix, press inward and feel as far as possible. Slide fingers so they are on top and bottom of cervix and continue pressing in while moving fingers to feel as much of uterus as possible. (When uterus is in midposition, you will not be able to feel it with outside hand.)

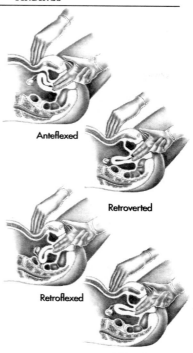

Anteflexed

Retroverted

Retroflexed

Midposition

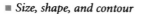

■ *Size, shape, and contour*

EXPECTED: Pear shaped and 5.5 to 8.0 cm long (larger in all dimensions in multiparous women). Contour rounded and, in nonpregnant women, walls firm and smooth.
UNEXPECTED: Larger than expected or interrupted contour or smoothness.

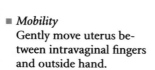

■ *Mobility*
Gently move uterus between intravaginal fingers and outside hand.

EXPECTED: Mobile in anteroposterior plane.
UNEXPECTED: Fixed uterus or tenderness on movement.

TECHNIQUE	FINDINGS

Palpate ovaries

Place fingers of outside hand on lower right quadrant. With intravaginal hand facing up, place both fingers in right lateral fornix. Press intravaginal fingers deeply in and up toward abdominal hand, while sweeping flat surface of fingers of outside hand deeply in and obliquely down toward symphysis pubis. Palpate entire area by firmly pressing outside hand and intravaginal fingers together.
Repeat on left side.

■ *Consistency*

EXPECTED: If palpable, ovaries should feel firm, smooth, and slightly to moderately tender.
UNEXPECTED: Marked tenderness or nodularity. Palpable fallopian tubes.

■ *Size*

EXPECTED: About 3 cm × 2 cm × 1 cm.
UNEXPECTED: Enlargement.

■ *Shape*

EXPECTED: Ovoid.

Palpate adnexal areas

Use hand positions for palpating ovaries.

EXPECTED: Adnexae difficult to palpate.
UNEXPECTED: Masses and tenderness. If adnexal masses are found, characterize by size, shape, location, consistency, and tenderness.

TECHNIQUE	FINDINGS

Internal Genitalia—Rectovaginal Examination

Change gloves.

This examination may be uncomfortable for the patient. Assure her that although she may feel the urgency of a bowel movement, she will not have one. Ask her to breathe slowly and try to relax her sphincter, rectum, and buttocks.

Insert index finger into vagina and middle finger into anus

To insert middle finger into anus, press against anus and ask patient to bear down. As she does, slip tip of finger into rectum just past sphincter.

Assess sphincter tone

Palpate area of anorectal junction and just above it. Ask patient to tighten and relax anal sphincter.

EXPECTED: Even sphincter tightening.
UNEXPECTED: Extremely tight, lax, or absent sphincter.

Palpate anterior rectal wall and rectovaginal septum

Slide both fingers in as far as possible, then ask patient to bear down. Rotate rectal finger to explore anterior rectal wall and palpate rectovaginal septum.

EXPECTED: Smooth and uninterrupted. Uterine body and uterine fundus sometimes felt with retroflexed uterus.
UNEXPECTED: Masses, polyps, nodules, strictures, and irregularities, and tenderness.

TECHNIQUE	FINDINGS

Palpate posterior aspect of uterus

Place outside hand just above symphysis pubis and press firmly and deeply down, while positioning intravaginal finger in posterior vaginal fornix and pressing strongly upward against posterior side of cervix, as shown in the figure at right. Palpate as much of posterior side of uterus as possible.

EXPECTED: Consistent with bimanual examination regarding location, position, size, shape, and contour.
UNEXPECTED: Tenderness.

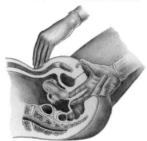

Palpate posterior rectal wall

As you withdraw fingers, rotate intrarectal finger to evaluate posterior rectal wall.

EXPECTED: Smooth and uninterrupted.
UNEXPECTED: Masses, polyps, nodules, strictures, irregularities, and tenderness.

Note characteristics of feces when gloved finger removed

EXPECTED: Light to dark brown in color.
UNEXPECTED: Blood. Note color of any blood and prepare specimen for fecal occult blood testing (FOBT).

Wipe patient's perineum, using front-to-back stroke and clean tissue for each stroke

AIDS TO DIFFERENTIAL DIAGNOSIS

ABNORMALITY	DESCRIPTION
Premenstrual syndrome (PMS)	Edema, headache, weight gain, and behavior disturbances such as irritability, nervousness, dysphoria, and lack of coordination. Symptoms occur 5 to 7 days before menses, then subside.
Endometriosis	Pelvic pain, dysmenorrhea, and heavy or prolonged menstrual flow.
Condyloma acuminatum (genital warts)	Warty lesions on labia, within vestibule, or in perianal region. The growths (generally whitish-pink to reddish-brown, discrete, and soft) may occur singly or in clusters, and may enlarge to cauliflower masses.
Herpes lesions	Small, red vesicles that may itch and usually are painful. Initial infection often extensive; recurrent infection normally a localized patch on vulva, perineum, vagina, or cervix.
Vaginal infections	Often vaginal discharge, possibly accompanied by urinary symptoms. Sometimes asymptomatic (see the table on pp. 182–183).
Cervical carcinoma	Hard granular surface at or near cervical os. Lesion can evolve to form extensive, irregular, easily bleeding cauliflower growth.
Uterine bleeding	See the table on p. 184.
Pelvic inflammatory disease (PID)	Acute PID: very tender bilateral adnexal areas. Chronic PID: bilateral tender, irregular, and fairly fixed adnexal areas.

Differential Diagnosis of Vaginal Discharges and Infections

CONDITION	HISTORY	PHYSICAL FINDINGS	DIAGNOSTIC TESTS
Physiologic vaginitis	Increase in discharge; no foul odor, itching, or edema	Clear or mucoid discharge; pH < 4.5	Wet mount: up to 3-5 white blood cells (WBCs); epithelial cells
Bacterial vaginosis (*Gardnerella vaginalis*)	Foul-smelling discharge; complains of "fishy odor"	Homogenous thin, white or gray discharge; pH > 4.5	+ KOH "whiff" test; Wet mount: + clue cells
Candida vulvovaginitis (*Candida albicans*)	Pruritic discharge; itching of labia; itching may extend to thighs	White, curdy discharge; pH 4.0-5.0; cervix may be red; may have erythema of perineum and thighs	KOH prep: mycelia, budding, branching yeast, pseudohyphae
Trichomoniasis (*Trichomonas vaginalis*)	Watery discharge; foul odor; dysuria, and dyspareunia with severe infection	Profuse, frothy, greenish discharge; pH 5.0-6.6; red friable cervix with petechiae ("strawberry" cervix)	Wet mount: round or pear-shaped protozoa, motile "gyrating" flagella
Gonorrhea (*Neisseria gonorrhoeae*)	Partner with sexually transmitted disease (STD); often asymptomatic or may have symptoms of pelvic inflammatory disease (PID)	Purulent discharge from cervix; Skene/Bartholin gland inflammation; cervix and vulva may be inflamed	Gram stain Culture DNA probe

Chlamydia (*Chlamydia trachomatis*)	Partner with nongonococcal urethritis; often asymptomatic; may complain of spotting after intercourse or urethritis	+/- purulent discharge; cervix may or may not be red or friable	DNA probe
Atrophic vaginitis	Dyspareunia; vaginal dryness; perimenopausal or postmenopausal	Pale thin vaginal mucosa; pH > 4.5	Wet mount: folded clumped epithelial cells
Allergic vaginitis	New bubble bath, soap, douche, or other hygiene products	Foul smell, erythema; pH < 4.5	Wet mount: WBCs
Foreign body	Red and swollen vulva; vaginal discharge; history of use of tampon, condom, or diaphragm	Bloody or foul-smelling discharge	Wet mount: WBCs

Bacterial vaginosis

Candida vulvovaginitis

Trichomoniasis

Types of Uterine Bleeding and Associated Causes	
TYPE	**COMMON CAUSES**
Midcycle spotting	Midcycle estradiol fluctuation associated with ovulation
Delayed menstruation with excessive bleeding	Anovulation or threatened abortion
Frequent bleeding	Chronic PID, endometriosis, DUB,* anovulation
Profuse menstrual bleeding	Endometrial polyps, DUB, adenomyosis, submucous leiomyomas, IUD
Intermenstrual or irregular bleeding	Endometrial polyps, DUB, uterine or cervical cancer, oral contraceptives
Postmenopausal bleeding	Endometrial hyperplasia, estrogen therapy, endometrial cancer

Modified from Thompson et al, 1997.
*DUB, Dysfunctional uterine bleeding.

PEDIATRIC VARIATIONS

EXAMINATION

TECHNIQUE	FINDINGS

External genitalia

Examine the infant using the frog-leg position.

EXPECTED: Genitalia of the newborn reflects the influence of maternal hormones. The labia majora and minora may be swollen, with the labia minora often more prominent.

Inspect clitoris

■ *Size and length*

EXPECTED: The clitoris of a term infant is usually covered by labia minora and may appear relatively large.

TECHNIQUE	FINDINGS

Inspect urethral meatus and vaginal opening

- *Inspect for discharge in infants and children*

EXPECTED: Mucoid whitish vaginal discharge is frequently seen during the newborn period and sometimes as late as 4 weeks after birth. The discharge may be mixed with blood.

UNEXPECTED: Mucoid discharge from irritation by diapers or powder; any discharge in children.

"Red Flags" for Sexual Abuse

The following signs and symptoms in children or adolescents should raise your suspicion for sexual abuse. Remember, however, that any sign or symptom by itself is of limited significance; it may be related to sexual abuse, or it may be from another cause altogether. This is an area in which good clinical judgment is imperative. Each sign or symptom must be considered in context with the particular child's health status, stage of growth and development, and entire history:

- Evidence of general physical abuse or neglect
- Evidence of trauma and/or scarring in genital, anal, and perianal areas
- Unusual changes in skin color or pigmentation in genital or anal area
- Presence of sexually transmitted disease (oral, anal, genital)
- Anorectal problems such as itching, bleeding, pain, fecal incontinence, poor anal sphincter tone, bowel habit dysfunction
- Genitourinary problems such as rash or sores in genital area, vaginal odor, pain (including abdominal pain), itching, bleeding, discharge, dysuria, hematuria, urinary tract infections, enuresis
- Behavioral manifestations such as use of sexually provocative mannerisms, excessive masturbation, unusual or inappropriate sexual knowledge or experience
- Significant behavioral changes such as problems with school, dramatic weight changes, depression

Modified from Koop CE, 1988.

External. Female hair distribution; no masses, lesions, or swelling. Urethral meatus intact without erythema or discharge. Perineum intact with healed episiotomy scar present. No lesions.

Internal. Vaginal mucosa moist and pink with rugae present. No unusual odors. Discharge scant and white. Cervix pink with horizontal slit, midline, no lesions or discharge.

Bimanual. Cervix smooth, firm, mobile, without motion tenderness. Uterus midline, anteverted, firm, smooth, nontender, not enlarged. Ovaries not palpable. No adnexal tenderness.

Rectovaginal. Sphincter tone intact; anal ring smooth and intact. Rectovaginal septum intact. No masses or tenderness. Stool brown; occult blood tested negative.

CHAPTER 14

MALE GENITALIA

EQUIPMENT

- Gloves

EXAMINATION

Have patient lying or standing to start the examination.

TECHNIQUE	FINDINGS
Wear gloves on both hands	
Inspect pubic hair	
■ *Characteristics*	**EXPECTED:** Coarser than scalp hair.
■ *Distribution*	**EXPECTED:** Male hair distribution. Abundant in pubic region, continuing around scrotum to anal orifice, and possibly continuing in narrowing midline to umbilicus. Penis without hair, scrotum with scant hair.

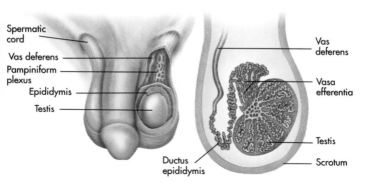

Spermatic cord
Vas deferens
Pampiniform plexus
Epididymis
Testis

Vas deferens
Vasa efferentia
Testis
Scrotum
Ductus epididymis

TECHNIQUE	FINDINGS

Inspect glans penis

- *Uncircumcised patient*
Retract foreskin.

EXPECTED: Dorsal vein apparent. Foreskin easily retracted. White, cheesy smegma visible over glans.
UNEXPECTED: Tight foreskin (phimosis). Lesions or discharge.

- *Circumcised patient*

EXPECTED: Dorsal vein apparent. Exposed glans erythematous and dry.
UNEXPECTED: Lesions or discharge.

Examine external meatus of urethra (foreskin retracted in uncircumcised patient)

- *Shape*

EXPECTED: Slitlike opening.
UNEXPECTED: Pinpoint or round opening.

- *Location*

EXPECTED: On ventral surface and only millimeters from tip of glans.
UNEXPECTED: Any place other than tip of glans or along shaft of penis.

- *Urethral orifice*
Press glans between thumb and forefinger.

EXPECTED: Opening glistening and pink.
UNEXPECTED: Bright erythema or discharge.

Palpate penis

EXPECTED: Soft (flaccid penis).
UNEXPECTED: Tenderness, induration, or nodularity. Prolonged erection (priapism).

TECHNIQUE	FINDINGS

Strip urethra

Firmly compress base of penis with thumb and forefinger; move toward glans.

UNEXPECTED: Discharge.

Inspect scrotum and ventral surface of penis

■ *Color*

EXPECTED: Darker than body skin and often reddened in red-haired patients.
UNEXPECTED: Reddened in patients without red hair.

■ *Texture*

EXPECTED: Surface possibly coarse. Small lumps on scrotal skin (sebaceous or epidermoid cysts) that sometimes discharge oily material.

■ *Shape*

EXPECTED: Asymmetry. Thickness varying with temperature, age, and emotional state.
UNEXPECTED: Unusual thickening, often with pitting.

Palpate inguinal canal for direct or indirect hernia

With patient standing, ask him to bear down as if for bowel movement. While he strains, inspect area of inguinal canal and region of fossa ovalis. Ask patient to relax, and insert examining finger into lower part of scrotum and carry upward along vas deferens into inguinal canal, as shown in the figure on p. 190. Ask patient to cough.

EXPECTED: Presence of oval external ring.
UNEXPECTED: Feeling a viscus against examining finger with coughing. If hernia felt, note as indirect (felt within inguinal canal or even into scrotum) or direct (felt medial to external canal).

TECHNIQUE	FINDINGS

Repeat examination on opposite side.

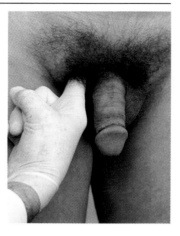

Palpate testes

Use thumb and first two fingers.

■ *Consistency*

EXPECTED: Smooth and rubbery. Sensitive to gentle compression.
UNEXPECTED: Tenderness or nodules. Total insensitivity to painful stimuli.

■ *Texture*

UNEXPECTED: Irregular texture.

■ *Size*

UNEXPECTED: Irregular size; asymmetry in size, less than 1 cm or greater than 5 cm.

■ *Descension*

Palpate epididymides

EXPECTED: Smooth and discrete, with the larger part cephalad.
UNEXPECTED: Tenderness.

TECHNIQUE	FINDINGS

Palpate vas deferens

Palpate from testicle to inguinal ring. Repeat with other testicle.

EXPECTED: Smooth and discrete.
UNEXPECTED: Beaded or lumpy.

Palpate for inguinal lymph nodes

Ask patient to lie supine, with knee slightly flexed on side of palpation.

EXPECTED: Nodes accessible to palpation, but not large enough or firm enough to be felt.
UNEXPECTED: Enlarged, tender, red or discolored, fixed, matted, inflamed, or warm nodes and increased vascularity.

Elicit cremasteric reflex bilaterally

Stroke inner thigh with blunt instrument. Repeat with other thigh.

EXPECTED: Testicle and scrotum on stroked side rise.

AIDS TO DIFFERENTIAL DIAGNOSIS

ABNORMALITY	DESCRIPTION
Herpes	Superficial vesicles—located on glans, penile shaft, or base of penis—that are frequently quite painful. Often associated with inguinal lymphadenopathy and systemic symptoms (e.g., fever) in primary infection.
Hernia	See the table on p. 192.
Hydrocele	Nontender, smooth, firm mass in scrotum. Transilluminates.
Varicocele	Abnormal tortuosity and dilated veins of pampiniform plexus within spermatic cord. Generally on left side and sometimes painful.

Distinguishing Characteristics of Hernias

	INDIRECT INGUINAL	DIRECT INGUINAL	FEMORAL
Incidence	Most common type of hernia; both sexes are affected; often patients are children and young males	Less common than indirect inguinal; occurs more often in males than females; more common in those over age 40	Least common type of hernia; occurs more often in females than males; rare in children
Occurrence	Through internal inguinal ring; can remain in canal, exit the external ring, or pass into scrotum; may be bilateral	Through external inguinal ring; located in region of Hesselbach triangle; rarely enters scrotum	Through femoral ring, femoral canal, and fossa ovalis
Presentation	Soft swelling in area of internal ring; pain on straining; hernia comes down canal and touches fingertip on examination	Bulge in area of Hesselbach triangle; usually painless; easily reduced; hernia bulges anteriorly; pushes against side of finger on examination	Right side presentation more common than left; pain may be severe; inguinal canal empty on examination

ABNORMALITY	DESCRIPTION
Epididymitis	Pain and possible erythema of overlying scrotum. Fever and white blood cells and bacteria in urine often accompany condition. In chronic form, epididymis feels firm and lumpy and may be slightly tender, and vasa deferentia may be beaded.
Priapism	Prolonged painful penile erection. Can occur in patients with leukemia or sickle cell disease.
Hypospadias	Urethral meatus is located on ventral surface of glans, penile shaft, or perineal area.
Epispadias	Urethral meatus is located on dorsal surface of the penile shaft.

PEDIATRIC VARIATIONS

EXAMINATION

TECHNIQUE	FINDINGS

Inspect Glans Penis

- *Uncircumcised patient* Retract foreskin.

EXPECTED: In children, the foreskin is fully retractable by age 3 to 4 years. Prior to that age, forced retraction of the foreskin may result in injury to the child.

Palpate scrotum

- *Descension* Palpate testes in children to determine if testes have descended. If any mass other than the testicles or spermatic cord is palpated in the scrotum, determine if it is filled with fluid, gas, or solid material.

EXPECTED: Bilaterally palpable; 1 cm in size. Considered descended if testis can be pushed into scrotum.
UNEXPECTED: If penlight transilluminates, then most likely contains fluid (hydrocele). If no light transillumination, then most likely a hernia.

Genitalia: Circumcised. Glans, penile shaft, and contents of the scrotal sac are intact without lesions or areas of induration. Urethral meatus patent on ventral surface at tip of glans. No discharge evident. Scrotal contents smooth without swelling, masses, or tenderness. Testes equal size. Inguinal areas are smooth, no masses or nodes palpable. Inguinal canals are free of masses, bulges. Cremasteric reflex elicited.

CHAPTER 15

ANUS, RECTUM, AND PROSTATE

EQUIPMENT

- Gloves
- Water-soluble lubricant
- Penlight
- Drapes
- Fecal occult blood testing materials

EXAMINATION

Have patient in knee-chest or left lateral position with hips and knees flexed, or standing with hips flexed and upper body supported by examining table. Drape patient appropriately.

TECHNIQUE	FINDINGS
Wear gloves on both hands	
Inspect and palpate sacrococcygeal and perianal area	
■ *Skin characteristics*	**EXPECTED:** Smooth and uninterrupted.
	UNEXPECTED: Lumps, rashes, tenderness, inflammation, excoriation, pilonidal dimpling, or tufts of hair.
Inspect anus	
Spread patient's buttocks. Examine, using penlight or lamp if needed, with patient relaxed as well as with patient bearing down.	
■ *Skin characteristics*	**EXPECTED:** Skin coarser and darker than on buttocks.

TECHNIQUE	FINDINGS

UNEXPECTED: Skin lesions, skin tags or warts, external or internal hemorrhoids, fissures, and fistulas, rectal prolapse, or polyps. Describe any irregularities and locate using clock referents (12 o'clock ventral midline/6 o'clock dorsal midline).

Inspect, palpate, and assess sphincter tone

Put water-soluble lubricant on index finger; press pad against anal opening and ask patient to bear down to relax external sphincter. As relaxation occurs, slip tip of finger into anal canal, as shown in the figure at right. (Assure patient that although he or she may feel the urgency of a bowel movement, it will not occur.) Ask patient to tighten external sphincter around finger.

EXPECTED: Even sphincter tightening.
UNEXPECTED: Patient discomfort. Lax or extremely tight sphincter, tenderness.

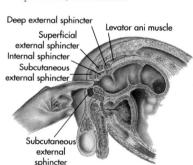

Deep external sphincter
Superficial external sphincter
Internal sphincter
Subcutaneous external sphincter
Levator ani muscle
Subcutaneous external sphincter

Palpate muscular anal ring

Rotate finger.

EXPECTED: Smooth and even with consistent pressure exerted.
UNEXPECTED: Nodules or other irregularities.

TECHNIQUE	FINDINGS

Palpate lateral and posterior rectal walls

Insert finger farther and rotate to palpate the lateral, then posterior, rectal walls. (If helpful, perform bidigital palpation with thumb and index finger by lightly pressing thumb against perianal tissue and bringing index finger toward thumb.)

EXPECTED: Smooth, even, and uninterrupted.
UNEXPECTED: Nodules, masses, polyps, tenderness, or irregularities. (Internal hemorrhoids not usually felt unless thrombosed.)

Males: Palpate posterior surface of prostate gland through anterior rectal wall

Rotate finger and palpate anterior rectal wall and the posterior surface of prostate gland. (Alert patient that he may feel urge to urinate but won't.)

■ *Consistency and characteristics of anterior rectal wall*

EXPECTED: Smooth, even, and uninterrupted.
UNEXPECTED: Nodules, masses, polyps, tenderness, or iregularities.

■ *Consistency, contour, and characteristics of prostate*

EXPECTED: Surface firm and smooth, lateral lobes symmetric, median sulcus palpable, and seminal vesicles not palpable.
UNEXPECTED: Rubberiness, bogginess, fluctuant softness, stony hard nodularity, tenderness, obliterated sulcus, or palpable seminal vesicles.

■ *Mobility of prostate gland*
■ *Size of prostate gland*

EXPECTED: Slightly movable.
EXPECTED: 4 cm diameter with less than 1 cm protruding into rectum.

TECHNIQUE   FINDINGS

UNEXPECTED: Protrusion
greater than 1 cm (note distance of protrusion).
UNEXPECTED: Discharge that
appears at urethral meatus (collect specimen for microscopic
examination).

Females: Palpate uterus through anterior rectal wall

Attempt to palpate uterus
and cervix through ante-
rior rectal wall.
- *Position*   **EXPECTED:** Midline,
                                  retroflexed or retroverted.
                                  UNEXPECTED: Deviation to
                                  right or left.
- *Surface characteristics*   **EXPECTED:** Smooth.
                                  UNEXPECTED: Irregular.

Have patient bear down, and palpate deeper

Ask patient to bear down   **UNEXPECTED:** Tenderness of
while you reach farther   peritoneal area or nodules.
into rectum. Females: ex-
plore in cul-de-sac. Males:
explore above prostate.

Withdraw finger and examine fecal material

- *Color and consistency*   **EXPECTED:** Soft and brown.
                                  UNEXPECTED: Blood, pus, or
                                  light-tan, gray, or tarry-black
                                  stool. Test any fecal material for
                                  blood using chemical fecal oc-
                                  cult blood testing (FOBT) pro-
                                  cedure

AIDS TO DIFFERENTIAL DIAGNOSIS

ABNORMALITY	DESCRIPTION
Perianal and perirectal abscesses	Pain and tenderness in anal area, usually accompanied by a fever.
Enterobiasis infestation in children	Intense perianal itching, especially at night.
Anorectal fissure and fistula	Fissure: Pain, itching, or bleeding, with spastic internal sphincter. Fistula: Elevated, red, granular tissue at external opening, possibly with serosanguinous or purulent drainage on compression of the area.
Hemorrhoids	External: Itching and bleeding with defecation. Thrombosed hemorrhoids appear as blue, shiny masses at anus. Internal: Bleeding with or without defecation. Do not cause discomfort unless thrombosed, prolapsed, or infected.
Rectal carcinoma	Generally asymptomatic.
Prostatic carcinoma	On rectal examination, a hard irregular nodule may be palpable. Prostate feels asymmetric and median sulcus is obliterated in advanced carcinoma.
Benign prostatic hypertrophy	Hesitancy on urination, decreased force and caliber of stream, dribbling, incomplete emptying of bladder, nocturia, and dysuria.

PEDIATRIC VARIATIONS

EXAMINATION

TECHNIQUE	FINDINGS
Inspect perianal area	
	UNEXPECTED: Parental complaints of infant's or child's irritability at night or evidence that child has itching in the perianal area may indicate the presence of parasites or round worms or pinworms. Specimen collection and microscopic examination is necessary to confirm findings.

SAMPLE DOCUMENTATION

Anus, rectum, prostate: Perianal area intact without lesions. An external skin tag is visible at 4 o'clock. No fissures or fistulas. Sphincter tone tightens evenly. Prostate is symmetrical, smooth, firm, nontender, without enlargement or nodules. Rectal walls free of masses. Moderate amount of soft stool present; occult blood test negative.

CHAPTER 16

MUSCULOSKELETAL SYSTEM

EQUIPMENT

- Goniometer
- Skin-marking pencil
- Reflex hammer
- Tape measure

EXAMINATION

Begin examination as patient enters rooms, observing gait and posture. During examination, note ease of movement when the patient walks, sits, rises, takes off garments, and responds to directions.

TECHNIQUE	FINDINGS

Posture and General Guidelines

Inspect skeleton and extremities, comparing sides

Inspect anterior, posterior, and lateral aspects of posture; ability to stand erect; body parts; and extremities.

- *Size, alignment, contour, and symmetry*
  Measure the extremities when lack of symmetry is noted in length or circumference

EXPECTED: Bilateral symmetry of length, circumference, alignment, and position and number of skin folds; symmetric body parts; and aligned extremities.

UNEXPECTED: Gross deformity, lordosis, kyphosis, scoliosis, bony enlargement.

TECHNIQUE	FINDINGS

Inspect skin and subcutaneous tissues over muscles, cartilage, bones, and joints

UNEXPECTED: Discoloration, swelling, or masses.

Inspect muscles and compare sides

■ *Size and symmetry*

EXPECTED: Approximately symmetric bilateral muscle size.
UNEXPECTED: Gross hypertrophy or atrophy, fasciculations, or spasms.

Palpate all bones, joints, and surrounding muscles (palpate inflamed joints last)

■ *Muscle tone*

EXPECTED: Firm.
UNEXPECTED: Hard or doughy.

■ *Characteristics*

UNEXPECTED: Heat, tenderness, swelling, fluctuation of a joint, synovial thickening, crepitus, resistance to pressure, or discomfort to pressure on bones and joints.

Test each major joint and related muscle groups for active and passive range of motion, and compare sides

Ask patient to move each joint through range of motion (see instructions for specific joints and muscles in individual sections that follow), then ask patient to relax as you passively move same joints until end of range is felt.

EXPECTED: Passive range of motion often exceeds active range of motion by 5 degrees. Range of motion with passive and active maneuvers should be equal between contralateral joints.

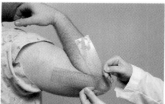

TECHNIQUE	FINDINGS

UNEXPECTED: Pain, limitation of motion, spastic movement, joint instability, deformity, contracture, and discrepancies greater than 5 degrees between active and passive range of motion. When increase or limitation in range of motion is found, measure angles of greatest flexion and extension with goniometer, as shown in the figure on p. 202, and compare with values as described for specific joints in individual sections.

Muscle Strength

MUSCLE FUNCTION LEVEL	SCALES		
	GRADE	% NORMAL	LOVETT SCALE
No evidence of contractility	0	0	0 (zero)
Slight contractility, no movement	1	10	T (trace)
Full range of motion, gravity eliminated*	2	25	P (poor)
Full range of motion against gravity	3	50	F (fair)
Full range of motion against gravity, some resistance	4	75	G (good)
Full range of motion against gravity, full resistance	5	100	N (normal)

From Barkauskas et al, 1998.
Passive movement.

TECHNIQUE	FINDINGS

Test major muscle groups for strength and compare contralateral sides

For each muscle group, ask patient to contract a muscle by flexing or extending a joint and resist as you apply opposing force. Compare bilaterally.

EXPECTED: Bilaterally symmetric with full resistance to opposition.
UNEXPECTED: Inability to produce full resistance. Grade muscular strength according to the table on p. 203.

Temporomandibular Joint

Palpate joint space for clicking, popping, and pain

Locate temporomandibular joints with fingertips placed just anterior to tragus of each ear, as shown in the figure at right. Ask patient to open mouth and allow fingertips to slip into joint space. Gently palpate.

EXPECTED: Audible or palpable snapping or clicking may be noted.
UNEXPECTED: Pain, crepitus, locking, or popping.

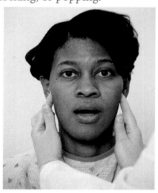

Test range of motion

Ask patient to:
■ *Open and close mouth*

EXPECTED: Opens 3 to 6 cm between upper and lower teeth.

■ *Move jaw laterally to each side*

EXPECTED: Mandible moves 1 to 2 cm in each direction.

TECHNIQUE	FINDINGS

■ *Protrude and retract jaw* **EXPECTED:** Both protrusion and retraction possible.

Test strength of temporalis and masseter muscles with patient's teeth clenched

Ask patient to clench teeth while you palpate contracted muscles and apply opposing force. (This also tests cranial nerve V motor function.)

EXPECTED: Bilaterally symmetric with full resistance to opposition.
UNEXPECTED: Inability to produce full resistance.

Cervical Spine

Inspect neck from anterior and posterior position

■ *Alignment* **EXPECTED:** Cervical spine straight, with head erect and in approximate alignment.

■ *Symmetry of skinfolds* **UNEXPECTED:** Asymmetric skinfolds.

Palpate posterior neck, cervical spine, and paravertebral, trapezius, and sternocleidomastoid muscles

EXPECTED: Good muscle tone, symmetry in size.
UNEXPECTED: Palpable tenderness or muscle spasm.

Test range of motion

■ *Forward flexion*
Bend head forward, chin to chest.

EXPECTED: 45-degree flexion.

■ *Hyperextension*
Bend head backward, chin toward ceiling.

EXPECTED: 45-degree hyperextension.

■ *Lateral bending*
Bend head to each side, ear to each shoulder.

EXPECTED: 40-degree lateral bending.

TECHNIQUE	FINDINGS

■ *Rotation*

Turn head to each side, chin to shoulder.

EXPECTED: 70-degree rotation.

Test strength of sternocleidomastoid and trapezius muscles

Ask patient to maintain each of the previous positions while you apply opposing force. (Cranial nerve XI is also tested with rotation.)

EXPECTED: Bilaterally symmetric strength with full resistance to opposition.
UNEXPECTED: Inability to produce full resistance.

Thoracic and Lumbar Spine

Inspect spine for alignment

Note major landmarks of back: each spinal process of vertebrae (C7 and T1 usually most prominent), scapulae, iliac crests, and paravertebral muscles.

EXPECTED: Head positioned directly over gluteal cleft, vertebrae straight (as indicated by symmetric shoulder, scapular, and iliac crest heights), curves of cervical and lumbar spines concave, curve of thoracic spine convex, and knees and feet aligned with trunk and pointing directly forward.
UNEXPECTED: Lordosis, kyphosis, scoliosis, or sharp angular deformity (gibbus).

Palpate spinal processes and paravertebral muscles

Ask patient to stand erect.

UNEXPECTED: Muscle spasm or spinal tenderness.

Percuss for spinal tenderness

Patient is still standing erect. First tap each spinal process with one finger, then rap each side of the spine along paravertebral muscles with ulnar aspect of fist.

UNEXPECTED: Muscle spasm or spinal tenderness.

TECHNIQUE	FINDINGS

Test range of motion and curvature

Ask patient to perform following movements (mark each spinal process with skin pencil if unexpected curvature suspected):

■ *Forward flexion*
Bend forward at waist and try to touch toes. Observe from behind to check curvature.

EXPECTED: 75- to 90-degree flexion, back remains symmetrically flat as concave curve of lumbar spine becomes convex with forward flexion.
UNEXPECTED: Lateral curvature or rib hump.

■ *Hyperextension*
Bend back at waist as far as possible.

EXPECTED: 30-degree hyperextension with reversal of lumbar curve.

■ *Lateral bending*
Bend to each side as far as possible.

EXPECTED: 35-degree lateral bending, each side.

■ *Rotation*
Swing upper trunk from waist in circular motion front to side to back to side while you stabilize pelvis.

EXPECTED: 30-degree rotation forward and backward.

Test for lumbar nerve root irritation (patient supine with neck slightly flexed)

■ *Straight leg raising test*
Ask patient to raise leg with knee extended. Repeat with other leg.

EXPECTED: No pain below knee with leg raising.
UNEXPECTED: Unable to raise leg more than 30 degrees without pain. Flexion of knee often eliminates pain with leg raising. Crossover pain in affected leg.

TECHNIQUE	FINDINGS

■ *Bragard stretch test*
Hold patient's lower leg
with the knee extended
and raise it slowly until
pain is felt. Lower the leg
slightly and briskly dorsiflex the foot.

UNEXPECTED: Pain with leg
raising and dorsiflexion.

Shoulders

Inspect shoulders, shoulder girdle, clavicles and scapulae,
and area muscles

■ *Size and contour*

EXPECTED: All shoulder
structures symmetric in size
and contour.
UNEXPECTED: Asymmetry,
hollows in the rounding contour, or winged scapula.

Palpate sternoclavicular and acromioclavicular joints,
clavicle, scapulae, coracoid process, greater trochanter of
humerus, biceps groove, and area muscles

EXPECTED: No tenderness or
masses, bilateral symmetry.
UNEXPECTED: Pain, tenderness, mass.

Test range of motion

Ask patient to perform
following movements:
■ *Shrug shoulders*
■ *Forward flexion*
Raise both arms forward
and straight up over head.
■ *Hyperextension*
Extend and stretch both
arms behind back.
■ *Abduction*
Lift both arms laterally
and straight up over head.

EXPECTED: Symmetric rising.

EXPECTED: 180-degree forward flexion.

EXPECTED: 50-degree hyperextension.

EXPECTED: 180-degree abduction.

TECHNIQUE   **FINDINGS**

- *Adduction*
  Swing each arm across the   **EXPECTED:** 50-degree adduc-
  front of the body.   tion.
- *Internal rotation*
  Place both arms behind   **EXPECTED:** 90-degree inter-
  hips, elbows out.   nal rotation.
- *External*
  Place both arms behind   **EXPECTED:** 90-degree exter-
  head, elbows out.   nal rotation.

Test shoulder girdle muscle strength

Ask patient to maintain
following positions while
you apply opposing force:
- *Shrugged shoulders*
  (This also tests cranial   **EXPECTED:** Bilaterally sym-
  nerve XI.)   metric with full resistance to
                                    opposition.
                                    UNEXPECTED: Inability to
                                    produce full resistance.

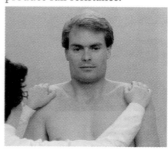

- *Forward flexion*   **EXPECTED:** Bilaterally sym-
                                    metric with full resistance to
                                    opposition.
                                    UNEXPECTED: Inability to
                                    produce full resistance.
- *Abduction*   **EXPECTED:** Bilaterally sym-
                                    metric with full resistance to
                                    opposition.

TECHNIQUE	FINDINGS

UNEXPECTED: Inability to produce full resistance.

Elbows

Inspect elbows in flexed and extended positions

- *Contour*

UNEXPECTED: Subcutaneous nodules along pressure points of extensor surface of ulna.

- *Carrying angle*
Inspect with arm passively extended, palm forward.

EXPECTED: Usually 5 to 15 degrees laterally.
UNEXPECTED: Lateral angle exceeding 15 degrees (cubitus valgus) or medial carrying angle (cubitus varus).

Palpate extensor surface of ulna, olecranon process, medial and lateral epicondyles of humerus, and groove on each side of olecranon process

Palpate with patient's elbow at 70 degrees.

UNEXPECTED: Boggy, soft, or fluctuant swelling; point tenderness at lateral epicondyle or along grooves of olecranon process and epicondyles.

Test range of motion

Ask patient to perform following movements:
- *Flexion and extension*
Bend and straighten elbow.

EXPECTED: 160-degree flexion from full extension at 0 degree.

- *Pronation and supination*
With elbow flexed at right angle, rotate hand from palm side down to palm side up.

EXPECTED: 90-degree pronation and 90-degree supination.
UNEXPECTED: Increased pain with pronation and supination of elbow.

TECHNIQUE	FINDINGS

Test muscle strength

Ask patient to maintain flexion and extension, as well as pronation and supination, while you apply opposing force.

EXPECTED: Bilaterally symmetric with full resistance to opposition.
UNEXPECTED: Inability to produce full resistance.

Hands and Wrists

Inspect dorsum and palm of each hand

■ *Characteristics and contour*

EXPECTED: Palmar and phalangeal creases. Palmar surfaces with central depression with prominent, rounded mound on thumb side (thenar eminence) and less prominent hypothenar eminence on little finger side.

■ *Position*

EXPECTED: Fingers able to fully extend and be aligned with forearm when in close approximation to each other.
UNEXPECTED: Deviation of fingers to ulnar side or swanneck or boutonnière deformities.

■ *Shape*

EXPECTED: Lateral finger surfaces gradually tapered from proximal to distal aspects.
UNEXPECTED: Spindleshaped fingers, bony overgrowths at phalangeal joints.

TECHNIQUE	FINDINGS

Palpate each joint in hand and wrist

Palpate interphalangeal joints with thumb and index finger, as shown in the figure at right; metacarpophalangeal joints with both thumbs, as shown in the figure below, left; and wrist and radiocarpal groove with thumbs on dorsal surface and fingers on palmar aspect of wrist, as shown in the figure below, right.

EXPECTED: Joint surfaces smooth.
UNEXPECTED: Nodules, swelling, bogginess, tenderness, or ganglion.

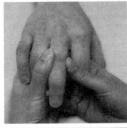

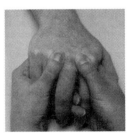

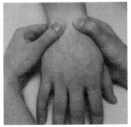

TECHNIQUE	FINDINGS

Strike median nerve for Tinel sign

Strike median nerve where it passes through carpal tunnel with index or middle finger.

UNEXPECTED: Tingling sensation radiating from wrist to hand along median nerve.

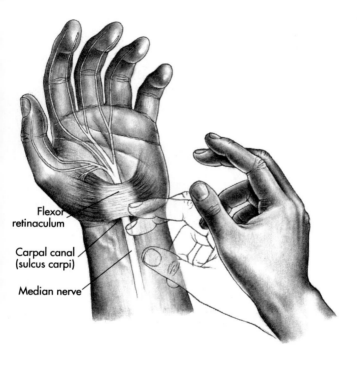

Flexor retinaculum

Carpal canal (sulcus carpi)

Median nerve

TECHNIQUE	FINDINGS

Test range of motion

Ask patient to perform following movements:

- *Metacarpophalangeal flexion and hyperextension*
Bend fingers forward at metacarpophalangeal joint, then stretch fingers up and back at knuckle.

EXPECTED: 90-degree metacarpophalangeal flexion and as much as 20-degree hyperextension.

- *Thumb opposition*
Touch thumb to each fingertip and to base of little finger, then make a fist.

EXPECTED: Able to perform all movements.

- *Finger abduction and adduction*
Spread fingers apart and then touch them together.

EXPECTED: Both movements possible.

- *Wrist extension and hyperextension*
Bend hand at wrist up and down.

EXPECTED: 90-degree flexion and 70-degree hyperextension.

- *Radial and ulnar motion*
With palm side down, turn each hand to right and left.

EXPECTED: 20-degree radial motion and 55-degree ulnar motion.

Test muscle strength

Ask patient to perform following movements:

- *Wrist extension and hyperextension*
Maintain wrist flexion while you apply opposing force.

EXPECTED: Bilaterally symmetric with full resistance to opposition.
UNEXPECTED: Inability to produce full resistance.

- *Hand strength*
Grip two of your fingers tightly.

EXPECTED: Firm, sustained grip.

TECHNIQUE	FINDINGS

UNEXPECTED: Weakness or pain.

Hips

Inspect hips for symmetry and level of gluteal folds

With patient standing, inspect anteriorly and posteriorly, using major landmarks of iliac crest and greater trochanter of femur.

UNEXPECTED: Asymmetry in iliac crest height, size of buttocks, or number and level of gluteal folds.

Palpate hips and pelvis

Have patient lie supine.

UNEXPECTED: Instability, tenderness, or crepitus.

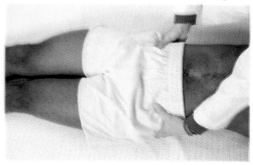

Test range of motion

While in position indicated, patient should perform following movements:

■ *Flexion, knee extended*
With patient supine, raise leg over body.

EXPECTED: Up to 90-degree flexion.

TECHNIQUE   FINDINGS

- *Hyperextension*
  While standing or prone,
  swing straightened leg behind body without arching
  the back.

  EXPECTED: Up to 30-degree
  hyperextension.

- *Flexion, knee flexed*
  While supine, raise one
  knee to chest while keeping other leg straight.

  EXPECTED: 120-degree flexion.

- *Abduction and adduction*
  While supine, swing leg
  laterally and medially with
  knee straight. During adduction movement, lift patient's opposite leg to
  permit examined leg full
  movement.

  EXPECTED: Up to 45-degree
  abduction and up to 30-degree
  adduction.

- *Internal rotation*
  While supine, flex knee
  and rotate leg inward toward other leg.

  EXPECTED: 40-degree internal rotation.

- *External rotation*
  While supine, place lateral
  aspect of foot on knee of
  other leg. Move flexed leg
  toward table.

  EXPECTED: 45-degree external rotation.

Test muscle strength

- *Knee in flexion and extension*
  Ask patient to maintain
  flexion of hip with knee in
  flexion and then extension
  while applying opposing
  force.

  EXPECTED: Bilaterally symmetric with full resistance to
  opposition.
  UNEXPECTED: Inability to
  produce full resistance.

- *Resistance to uncrossing the
  legs while seated.*

  EXPECTED: Bilaterally symmetric with full resistance to
  opposition.

TECHNIQUE	FINDINGS

Perform Thomas test to inspect for flexion contractures

While supine, patient should fully extend one leg flat on examining table and flex other leg with knee to chest.

EXPECTED: Patient able to keep extended leg flat on table.
UNEXPECTED: Extended leg lifts off table.

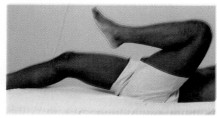

Perform Trendelenburg test to inspect for weak hip abductor muscles

Ask patient to stand and balance first on one foot, then the other. Observe from behind.

UNEXPECTED: Asymmetry or change in level of iliac crests.

Legs and Knees

Inspect knees and popliteal spaces, flexed and extended

Note major landmarks: tibial tuberosity, medial and lateral tibial condyles, medial and lateral epicondyles of femur, adductor tubercle of femur, and patella.

EXPECTED: Natural concavities on anterior aspect, on each side, and above patella.
UNEXPECTED: Usual indentation above patella is convex rather than concave.

Observe lower leg alignment

EXPECTED: Angle between femur and tibia less than 15 degrees. Bowlegs is a common finding until 18 months of age; knock knees is common between 2 and 4 years.

TECHNIQUE	FINDINGS

UNEXPECTED: Knock knees (genu valgum), bowlegs (genu varum), and excessive hyperextension of knee with weight bearing (genu recurvatum).

Palpate popliteal space

UNEXPECTED: Swelling or tenderness.

Palpate tibiofemoral joint space

Identify patella, suprapatellar pouch, and infrapatellar fat pad.

EXPECTED: Smooth and firm.
UNEXPECTED: Tenderness, bogginess, nodules, or crepitus.

Test range of motion

- *Flexion*
  Ask patient to bend each knee.

EXPECTED: 130-degree flexion.

- *Extension*
  Ask patient to straighten leg and stretch it.

EXPECTED: Full extension and up to 15-degree hyperextension.

Test muscle strength

- *Flexion and extension*
  Ask patient to maintain flexion and extension while you apply opposing force.

EXPECTED: Bilaterally symmetric with full resistance to opposition.
UNEXPECTED: Inability to produce full resistance.

TECHNIQUE   **FINDINGS**

Additional Techniques for Knees

Perform ballottement procedure to determine presence of excess fluid or an effusion in knee

With knee extended, apply downward pressure on suprapatellar pouch with thumb and fingers of one hand, then push the patella sharply backward against femur with finger of other hand, as shown at right. Suddenly release pressure on patella, while keeping finger lightly on knee.

UNEXPECTED: A tapping or clicking is sensed when patella is pushed against the femur. Patella then floats out as if a fluid wave is pushing it.

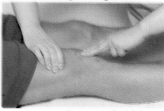

Test for bulge sign to determine presence of excess fluid in knee

With knee extended, milk medial aspect of knee upward two or three times, as shown below, then tap lateral side of patella, as shown below, right.

UNEXPECTED: Bulge of returning fluid to hollow area medial to patella.

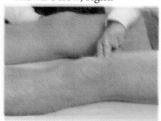

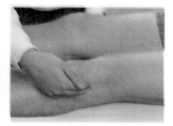

TECHNIQUE	FINDINGS

Perform McMurray test to detect torn meniscus

Ask patient to lie supine and flex one knee completely with foot flat on table near buttocks. Maintain that flexion with your thumb and index finger, while stabilizing knee. Hold heel with other hand, rotate foot and lower leg to lateral position, and extend knee to 90-degree angle. Return knee to full flexion, then rotate foot and lower leg to medial position, and extend knee to 90-degree angle.

UNEXPECTED: Palpable or audible click or limited extension of knee with either procedure.

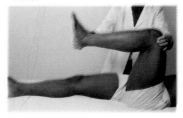

Perform drawer test to identify anteroposterior instability of knee

Ask patient to flex knee 45 to 90 degrees, placing foot flat on table. While stabilizing foot with one hand and grasping lower leg just below knee with other, try to push lower leg forward and pull backward.

UNEXPECTED: Anterior or posterior movement.

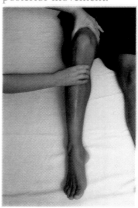

TECHNIQUE	FINDINGS

Perform varus valgus stress test to identify mediolateral instability of knee

Ask patient to lie supine and extend knee. While you stabilize femur with one hand and hold ankle with other, try to abduct and adduct knee. Repeat with knee flexed to 30 degrees.

UNEXPECTED: Excessive laxity, medial or lateral movement.

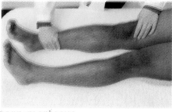

Perform Apley test to detect torn meniscus

Ask patient to lie prone and flex knee to 90 degrees. Place hand on heel of foot and press firmly, opposing tibia to femur. Carefully rotate lower leg externally and internally. Do not cause excess pain.

UNEXPECTED: Clicks, locking, or pain.

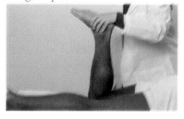

Feet and Ankles

Inspect during weight bearing (standing and walking) and nonweight bearing

Note major landmarks: medial malleolus, lateral malleolus, and Achilles tendon.

■ *Characteristics*

EXPECTED: Smooth and rounded malleolar prominence, prominent heels, and prominent metatarsophalangeal joints.

UNEXPECTED: Calluses and corns.

TECHNIQUE	FINDINGS
■ *Alignment*	**EXPECTED:** Feet aligned with tibias and weight bearing on foot midline. **UNEXPECTED:** In-toeing (pes varus), outtoeing (pes valgus), deviations in forefoot alignment (metatarsus varus or metatarsus valgus), heel pronation, or pain.
■ *Contour*	**EXPECTED:** Longitudinal arch that may flatten with weight bearing. Foot flat when not bearing weight (pes planus) and high instep (pes cavus) are common variations. **UNEXPECTED:** Pain with pes planus.
■ *Toes*	**EXPECTED:** Toes on each foot straight forward, flat, and in alignment. **UNEXPECTED:** Hammer toe; claw toe; mallet toe; hallux valgus; bunions, or heat, redness, swelling, and tenderness of the metatarsophalangeal joint of great toe (possibly with draining tophus).

Palpate Achilles tendon and each metatarsal joint

Using thumb and fingers of both hands, compress forefoot, palpating each metatarsophalangeal joint.	**EXPECTED:** No tenderness or masses, bilateral symmetry. **UNEXPECTED:** Pain, masses, thickened Achilles tendon.

TECHNIQUE	FINDINGS

Test range of motion

Ask patient to sit then perform following move-
ments:

■ *Dorsiflexion*
Point foot toward ceiling.

EXPECTED: 20-degree dorsiflexion.

■ *Plantar flexion*
Point foot toward floor.

EXPECTED: 45-degree plantar
flexion.

■ *Inversion and eversion*
Bend foot at ankle, then
turn sole of foot toward
and away from other foot.

EXPECTED: 30-degree inversion and 20-degree eversion.

■ *Abduction and adduction*
Rotate ankle, turning away
from and then toward
other foot (while you stabilize leg).

EXPECTED: 10-degree abduction and 20-degree adduction.

■ *Flexion and extension*
Bend and straighten toes.

EXPECTED: Some flexion and
extension, especially great toes.

Test strength of ankle muscles

Ask patient to maintain
dorsiflexion and plantar
flexion while you apply
opposing force.

EXPECTED: Bilaterally symmetric with full resistance to
opposition.
UNEXPECTED: Inability to
produce full resistance.

AIDS TO DIFFERENTIAL DIAGNOSIS

ABNORMALITY	DESCRIPTION
Carpal tunnel syndrome	Numbness, burning, and tingling in hands, often occurring at night but also elicited by rotational movement of wrist. Pain in arms. Can result in weakness of hand and flattening of the thenar eminence of palm.
Gout	Red, hot, swollen joint (classically the proximal phalanx of great toe, although other joints of wrist, hands, ankles, and knees are sometimes affected); exquisite pain; limited range of motion; tophi; and mild fever.
Lumbar disk herniation	Lower back pain with radiation to buttocks and posterior thigh or down leg in distribution of nerve root dermatome (see pp. 238-239), tenderness over paraspinal muscles, unilateral or bilateral pain, muscle weakness, paresthesia.
Bursitis	Motion limitation caused by swelling, pain on movement, point tenderness, erythema, and warmth; commonly occurs in shoulder, elbow, hip, and knee.
Osteoarthritis	See the table on p. 225.
Rheumatoid arthritis	See the table on p. 225.
Sprain	Pain, marked swelling, hemorrhage, and loss of function.
Fracture	Deformity, edema, pain, loss of function, color changes, and paresthesia.
Tenosynovitis	Point tenderness, edema, pain with movement, and weakness, commonly of shoulder, knee, heel, and wrist.

Differential Diagnosis of Arthritis

SIGNS AND SYMPTOMS	OSTEOARTHRITIS	RHEUMATOID ARTHRITIS
Onset	Insidious	Gradual or sudden (24-48 hr)
Duration of stiffness	Few minutes, localized, but short "gelling" after prolonged rest	Often hours, most pronounced after rest
Pain	On motion, with prolonged activity, relieved by rest	Even at rest, may disturb sleep
Weakness	Usually localized and not severe	Often pronounced, out of proportion with muscle atrophy
Fatigue	Unusual	Often severe, with onset 4-5 hr after rising
Emotional depression and lability	Unusual	Common, coincides with fatigue and disease activity, often relieved if in remission
Tenderness localized over afflicted joint	Common	Almost always, most sensitive indicator of inflammation
Swelling	Effusion common, little synovial reaction	Fusiform soft tissue enlargement, effusion common, synovial proliferation and thickening
Heat, erythema	Unusual	Sometimes present
Crepitus, crackling	Coarse to medium on motion	Medium to fine
Joint enlargement	Mild with firm consistency	Moderate to severe

Modified from McCarty, 1993.

ABNORMALITY	DESCRIPTION
Scoliosis	Uneven shoulder and hip levels, a rib hump, and flank asymmetry on forward flexion. Lateral curvature of spine resulting from leg length discrepancy also possible.
Osteoporosis	Height loss, bent spine, and the appearance of sinking into hips—most often in postmenopausal women. Usual presenting symptom is acute, painful fracture, most commonly of hip, vertebra, or wrist.

PEDIATRIC VARIATIONS

EXAMINATION

Musculoskeletal findings and motor development in the infant, child, and adolescent change as the child grows. For a complete description of age-specific anticipated pediatric findings, see Chapter 20.

Sports Participation Screening Examination for Children and Adolescents

- Observe posture and general muscle contour bilaterally.
- Observe gait.
- Ask patient to walk on tiptoes and heels.
- Observe patient hop on each foot.
- Ask patient to duck walk four steps with knees completely bent.
- Inspect spine for curvature and lumbar extension, fingers touching toes with knees straight.
- Palpate shoulder and clavicle for dislocation.
- Check the following for range of motion: neck, shoulder, elbow, forearm, hands, fingers, and hips.
- Test knee ligaments for drawer sign.

SAMPLE DOCUMENTATION

Posture erect and spine straight, without obvious deformities; muscles and extremities symmetric; muscle strength appropriate and equal bilaterally; active range of motion without pain, locking, clicking, or limitation in all joints.

CHAPTER 17

NEUROLOGIC SYSTEM

EQUIPMENT

- Familiar objects (coins, keys, paper clip)
- Vials of aromatic substances (coffee, orange, peppermint, banana)
- Sterile needles
- Cotton wisp
- Tongue blades (one intact and one broken with point and rounded edges)
- List of tastes
- Vials of solutions (glucose, salt, lemon or vinegar, and quinine) with applicators
- Cup of water
- Test tubes of hot and cold water
- Tuning forks
- Reflex hammer
- 5.07 monofilament

EXAMINATION

Evaluate the neurologic system as the rest of the body is examined. When history and examination findings have not revealed a potential neurologic problem, perform a neurologic screening examination as shown in the box on p. 228, rather than a full neurologic examination. See Chapter 16, Musculoskeletal System, for evaluation of muscle tone and strength.

Cranial Nerves I-XII

The table on pp. 230-231 summarizes the cranial nerve examination. When a sensory or motor loss is suspected, be compulsive about determining the extent of the loss.

Neurologic Screening Examination

This shorter screening examination is commonly used for health visits when no known neurologic problem is apparent.

CRANIAL NERVES

Cranial nerves II through XII are routinely tested; however, taste and smell are not tested unless some aberration is found.

PROPRIOCEPTION AND CEREBELLAR FUNCTION

One test is administered for each of the following: rapid rhythmic alternating movements, accuracy of movements, balance (Romberg test), and gait and heel-toe walking.

SENSORY FUNCTION

Superficial pain and touch at a distal point in each extremity are tested; vibration and position senses are assessed by testing the great toe.

DEEP TENDON REFLEXES

All deep tendon reflexes and the plantar reflex are tested, excluding the test for clonus.

TECHNIQUE   **FINDINGS**

Assess olfactory nerve (CN I)

Ask patient to close eyes. Occlude one naris, hold vial (using least irritating aromatic substances first, e.g., orange or peppermint extract) under nose, and ask patient to breathe deeply and identify odor. Allow patient to breathe comfortably, then occlude other naris and repeat with different odor. Continue, alternating two or three odors.

EXPECTED: Able to perceive and usually identify odor on each side.
UNEXPECTED: Anosmia, loss of smell or inability to discriminate odors.

Assess optic nerve (CN II)

See tests for visual acuity and visual fields in Chapter 7, Eyes.

TECHNIQUE	FINDINGS

Assess oculomotor, trochlear, and abducens nerves (CN III, CN IV, and CN VI)

See tests for six cardinal points of gaze, pupil size, shape, response to light and accommodation, and opening of upper eyelids in Chapter 7, Eyes.

EXPECTED: Equal pupil size, equal and consensual response to light and accommodation, symmetric eye movements in all six cardinal points of gaze.
UNEXPECTED: Absence of lateral gaze. Absence of any expected findings, ptosis.

Assess trigeminal nerve (CN V)

■ *Facial muscle tone*
Ask patient to clench teeth tightly as you palpate muscles over jaw.

EXPECTED: Symmetric tone.
UNEXPECTED: Muscle atrophy, deviation of jaw to one side, or fasciculations.

■ *Sensation*
Ask patient to close eyes and report if sensation to touch is present or is sharp or dull as you touch each side of face at scalp, cheek, and chin areas, alternately using sharp and rounded edges of tongue blades or paper clip, in an unpredictable pattern. Ask patient to report when the stimulus is felt as you stroke same six areas with cotton wisp or brush. Finally, test sensation over buccal mucosa with wooden applicator.

EXPECTED: Symmetric discrimination of sensations in each location to all stimuli.
UNEXPECTED: Impaired sensation. If impaired, use test tubes of hot and cold water to evaluate temperature sensation.

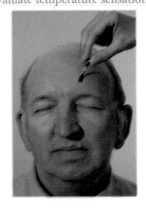

■ *Corneal reflex*
See test for corneal sensitivity in Chapter 7, Eyes.

Procedures for Cranial Nerve Examination

CRANIAL NERVE (CN)	PROCEDURE
CN I (Olfactory)	Test ability to identify familiar aromatic odors, one naris at a time with eyes closed.
CN II (Optic)	Test vision with Snellen chart and Rosenbaum near-vision chart. Perform ophthalmoscopic examination of fundi. Test visual fields by confrontation and extinction of vision.
CN III, IV, and VI (Oculomotor, trochlear, and abducens)	Test extraocular movement. Inspect eyelids for drooping. Inspect pupils' size for equality and their direct and consensual response to light and accommodation.
CN V (Trigeminal)	Inspect face for muscle atrophy and tremors. Palpate jaw muscles for tone and strength when patient clenches teeth. Test superficial pain and touch sensation in each branch. (Test temperature sensation if there are unexpected findings to pain or touch.) Test corneal reflex.
CN VII (Facial)	Inspect symmetry of facial features with various expressions (e.g., smile, frown, puffed cheeks, wrinkled forehead). Test ability to identify sweet and salty tastes on each side of tongue.

CN VIII (Acoustic)	Test sense of hearing with whisper screening tests or by audiometry.
	Compare bone and air conduction of sound.
	Test for lateralization of sound.
CN IX (Glossopharyngeal)	Test ability to identify sour and bitter tastes.
	Test gag reflex and ability to swallow.
CN X (Vagus)	Inspect palate and uvula for symmetry with speech sounds and gag reflex.
	Observe for swallowing difficulty.
	Evaluate quality of guttural speech sounds (presence of nasal or hoarse quality to voice).
CN XI (Spinal accessory)	Test trapezius muscle strength (shrug shoulders against resistance).
	Test sternocleidomastoid muscle strength (turn head to each side against resistance).
CN XII (Hypoglossal)	Inspect tongue in mouth and while protruded for symmetry, tremors, and atrophy.
	Inspect tongue movement toward nose and chin.
	Test tongue strength with index finger when tongue is pressed against cheek.
	Evaluate quality of lingual speech sounds (*l, t, d, n*).

TECHNIQUE	FINDINGS

Assess facial nerve (CN VII)

■ *Expressions*
Ask patient to make following facial expressions:
- Raise eyebrows and wrinkle forehead
- Smile
- Frown
- Puff out cheeks
- Purse lips and blow out
- Show teeth
- Squeeze eyes shut against resistance

EXPECTED: Facial symmetry.
UNEXPECTED: Tics, unusual facial movements, or asymmetry of expression (flattened nasolabial fold, lower eyelid sagging, side of mouth droops).

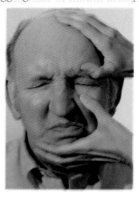

■ *Speech*

UNEXPECTED: Difficulties with enunciating *b*, *m*, and *p* (labial sounds).

■ *Taste (CN VII and CN IX)*
Hold card listing tastes in patient's view. Ask patient to extend tongue. Apply one of four solutions to lateral side of tongue in appropriate taste-bud region. Ask patient to point to taste perceived. Offer patient a sip of water and repeat with different solution and applicator, testing each side of tongue with each solution.

EXPECTED: Able to identify sweet, salt, sour, and bitter taste bilaterally when placed in appropriate taste-bud region.

TECHNIQUE	FINDINGS

Assess acoustic nerve (CN VIII)

See screening tests in Chapter 8, Ears, Nose, and Throat.

Assess glossopharyngeal nerve (CN IX)

■ *Taste*
See previous information regarding taste.
■ *Gag reflex (nasopharyngeal sensation)*
See following step for vagus nerve.

Assess vagus nerve (CN X)

■ *Gag reflex* (nasopharyngeal sensation) (CN IX and CN X)
Tell patient you will be testing gag reflex. Touch posterior wall of pharynx with applicator while observing palate, pharyngeal muscles, and uvula.

EXPECTED: Upward movement of palate and contraction of pharyngeal muscles, with uvula in midline.
UNEXPECTED: Drooping or absence of arch on either side of soft palate, uvula deviates from midline.

■ *Motor function*
Ask patient to say "ah" while observing movement of soft palate and uvula.

UNEXPECTED: Failure of soft palate to rise or deviation of uvula from midline.

■ *Swallowing (CN IX and CN X)*
Ask patient to swallow water.
■ *Speech*

EXPECTED: Water easily swallowed.
UNEXPECTED: Retrograde passage of water through nose.
UNEXPECTED: Hoarseness, nasal quality, or difficulty with guttural sounds.

TECHNIQUE	FINDINGS

Assess spinal accessory nerve (CN XI)

See Chapter 6, Head and Neck, and Chapter 16, Musculoskeletal System, for evaluations of the size, shape, and strength of the trapezius and sternocleidomastoid muscles.

Assess hypoglossal nerve (XII)

■ *Tongue resting and protruded*

Inspect while at rest on floor of mouth and while protruded.

EXPECTED: Tongue midline, symmetric size.

UNEXPECTED: Fasciculations, asymmetry, atrophy, or deviation from midline.

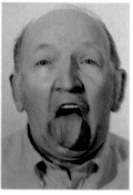

■ *Tongue movement*

Ask patient to move tongue in and out, side to side, curled up toward nose, and curled down toward chin.

EXPECTED: Able to perform most tongue movements.

■ *Tongue strength*

Ask patient to push tongue against cheek while you apply resistance with index finger.

EXPECTED: Steady, firm pressure.

TECHNIQUE	FINDINGS

■ *Speech*

UNEXPECTED: Problems with *l*, *t*, *d*, or *n* (lingual sounds).

Proprioception and Cerebellar Function

Evaluate coordination and fine motor skills

Have patient sit.

■ *Rapid, rhythmic, alternating movements*

Ask patient to pat knees with both hands, alternately patting with palms then backs of the hands. Alternatively, ask the patient to touch the thumb to each finger of the same hand sequentially from index finger to little finger and back; one hand at a time.

EXPECTED: Smooth execution, maintaining rhythm with increasing speed.

UNEXPECTED: Stiff, slowed, nonrhythmic, or jerky clonic movements.

■ *Accuracy of movement: finger-to-finger test*

Position your index finger 40 to 50 cm from patient. Ask patient to alternately touch his or her nose and your index finger with the index finger of one hand, as shown at right. Change location of your index finger several times. Repeat with patient's other hand.

EXPECTED: Movements rapid, smooth, and accurate.

UNEXPECTED: Consistent past pointing.

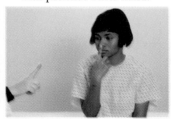
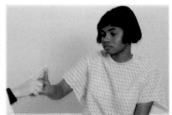

TECHNIQUE	FINDINGS

■ *Accuracy of movement: finger-to-nose test*
Ask patient to close both eyes and touch his or her nose with index finger of each hand while alternating hands and gradually increasing speed.

EXPECTED: Movements rapid, smooth, and accurate, even with increasing speed.

■ *Accuracy of movement: heel-to-shin test* (can be performed sitting, standing or supine)
Ask patient to run heel of one foot along shin from knee to ankle of opposite leg. Repeat with other heel.

EXPECTED: Able to move heel up and down shin in straight line.
UNEXPECTED: Irregular deviations to side.

Evaluate balance

■ *Balance: Romberg test*
Ask patient to stand with feet together and arms at sides, first with eyes open, then closed. ***Stand close by in case patient starts to fall.***

EXPECTED: Slight swaying movement, no danger of falling.
UNEXPECTED: Staggering, losing balance, or swaying to the extent of falling.

■ *Balance: recovery*
After explaining test to patient, ask patient to spread feet slightly, then push shoulders to throw her or him off balance. ***Be prepared to catch patient.***

EXPECTED: Quick recovery of balance.
UNEXPECTED: Must catch patient to prevent a fall.

■ *Balance: standing and hopping*
Have patient stand in place on one foot, then the other, with eyes open. Then have patient hop on each foot.

EXPECTED: Able to stand and hop 5 seconds on each foot without losing balance.
UNEXPECTED: Instability, need to continually touch floor with opposite foot, or tendency to fall.

TECHNIQUE	FINDINGS

■ *Gait: walking*
Ask patient to walk without shoes around examining room or down hallway, first with eyes open, then closed.

EXPECTED: Smooth, regular gait rhythm and symmetric stride length; upright trunk posture swaying with gait phase; and arm swing smooth and symmetric.
UNEXPECTED: Shuffling, widely placed feet, toe walking, foot flop, leg lag, scissoring, loss of arm swing, staggering, lurching, or waddling motion.

■ *Gait: straight-line walking*
Ask patient to walk a straight line, first forward and then backward, with eyes open and arms at side. Ask patient to touch toe of one foot with heel of other.

EXPECTED: Consistent contact between toe and heel with slight swaying.
UNEXPECTED: Extension of arms for balance, instability, tendency to fall, or lateral staggering and reeling.

Sensory Function

Test primary sensory functions
Ask patient to close eyes for all tests. Use minimal stimulation initially, then increase gradually until patient becomes aware. Test contralateral areas, asking patient to compare perceived sensations side to side.

EXPECTED: *For all tests, minimal differences side to side, correct interpretation of sensations, discrimination of side of body tested, and location of sensation (e.g., proximal or distal to previous stimulus).*
UNEXPECTED: *For all tests,* map boundaries of any impairment by distribution of major peripheral nerves or dermatomes (see figures on pp. 238-239).

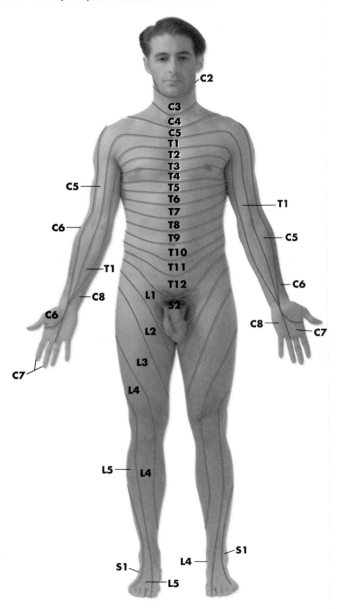

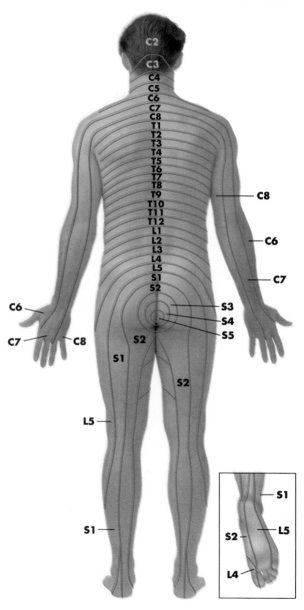

TECHNIQUE	FINDINGS

- *Superficial touch*
  Lightly touch skin with cotton wisp or your fingertips, as shown at right. Ask patient to point to area touched or acknowledge when sensation is felt.

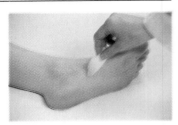

- *Superficial pain*
  Alternating sharp and smooth edge of broken tongue blade or point and hub of sterile needle, touch skin in unpredictable pattern. Ask patient to identify sensation (sharp or dull) and where it is felt.

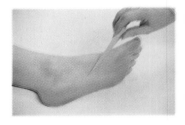

- *Temperature and deep pressure*
  Necessary to perform test only if superficial pain sensation is not intact.
  Temperature: Alternately roll test tubes of hot and cold water against skin in an unpredictable pattern. Ask patient to indicate hot or cold and where it is felt.
  Deep pressure: Squeeze trapezius, calf, or biceps muscle.

EXPECTED: Discomfort with deep pressure.

TECHNIQUE   **FINDINGS**

- *Protective sensation*
  Necessary to perform test only if patient has diabetes mellitus or peripheral neuropathy.
  Apply a 5.07 monofilament in a random pattern to several sites on the plantar surface of the foot and once on dorsal surface until filament bends. Avoid calloused areas and broken skin.

EXPECTED: Sensation felt at all sites touched.
UNEXPECTED: Loss of sensation at any site.

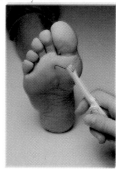

- *Vibration*
  Place stem of vibrating tuning fork against several bony prominences (e.g., toes, ankle, shin, finger joints, wrist, elbow, shoulder, and sternum), beginning distally. Ask patient when and where sensation is felt and what it feels like. Dampen the tines occasionally to see if patient notices difference.

EXPECTED: Buzzing or tingling sensation.
UNEXPECTED: Does not distinguish vibration from touch of tuning fork.

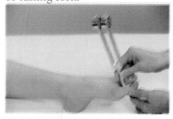

- *Position of joints*
  Hold joint to be tested (great toe or finger) by lateral aspects in neutral position, then raise or lower digit, as shown, and ask patient which way it was moved. Return to neutral before moving in another direction. Repeat so both feet and both hands are tested.

EXPECTED: Patient correctly identifies position of joint.

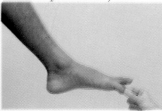

TECHNIQUE	FINDINGS

Test cortical sensory functions.

Ask patient to close eyes
for all tests.

■ *Stereognosis*
Hand patient familiar ob-
jects (e.g., key, coin), and
ask patient to identify.

UNEXPECTED: Inability to
recognize objects (tactile ag-
nosia).

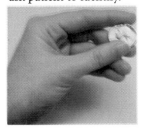

■ *Two-point discrimination*
Using two sterile needles,
alternately touch patient's
skin with one point or
both points simultane-
ously at various locations.
Find distance at which patient can no longer distinguish two points.

EXPECTED: See the table on
p. 243.

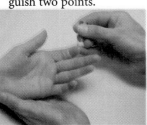

Minimal Distances of Discriminating Two Points	
BODY PART	**MINIMAL DISTANCE (MM)**
Tongue	1
Fingertips	2-8
Toes	3-8
Palms of hands	8-12
Chest and forearms	40
Back	40-70
Upper arms and thighs	75

From Barkauskas et al, 1998.

TECHNIQUE	FINDINGS

- *Extinction phenomenon*
  Simultaneously touch cheek, hand, or other area on each side of body with sterile needles. Ask patient the number of stimuli and locations.

  EXPECTED: Both sensations felt.

- *Graphesthesia*
  With blunt pen or applicator stick, draw letter or number on palm of patient's hand, and ask patient to identify it. Repeat with different figure on other hand.

  EXPECTED: Letter or number readily recognized.

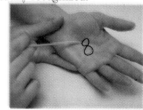

- *Point location*
  Touch area on patient's skin and withdraw stimulus. Ask patient to point to area touched.

  EXPECTED: Able to locate stimulus.

TECHNIQUE	FINDINGS

Reflexes

Test superficial reflexes

Have patient supine.
- *Abdominal*
  Stroke each quadrant of abdomen with end of reflex hammer or with tongue blade edge.

EXPECTED: Slight, bilaterally equal movement of umbilicus toward each area of stimulation.

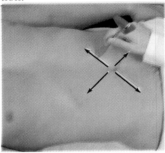

- *Cremasteric (male patients)*
  Stroke inner thigh, proximal to distal.

EXPECTED: Testicle and scrotum rise on stroked side.

- *Plantar reflex*
  Using pointed object, stroke lateral side of foot from heel to ball, then curve across ball to medial side.

EXPECTED: Plantar flexion of all toes.

UNEXPECTED: Fanning of toes or dorsiflexion of great toe with or without fanning of other toes (Babinski sign).

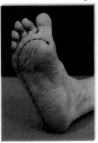

TECHNIQUE	FINDINGS

Test deep tendon reflexes

Patient relaxed and either sitting or lying for most procedures. Test each reflex, comparing responses on corresponding sides. Score the deep tendon reflexes on scale shown in the table on p. 246.

EXPECTED: Symmetric visible or palpable responses.
UNEXPECTED: Absent or diminished responses (0 or 1+), or hyperactive reflexes (3+ or 4+).

■ *Biceps*
Flex arm up 45 degrees at elbow, then palpate biceps tendon in antecubital fossa. Place thumb over tendon and fingers under the elbow. Strike your thumb with reflex hammer.

EXPECTED: Visible or palpable flexion of elbow, contraction of biceps muscle.

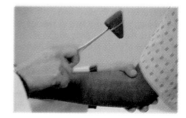

■ *Brachioradial*
Flex patient's arm up to 45 degrees while resting patient's forearm on your arm, with hand slightly pronated. Strike brachioradial tendon.

EXPECTED: Pronation of forearm and flexion of elbow.

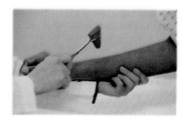

Scoring Deep Tendon Reflexes	
GRADE	DEEP TENDON REFLEX RESPONSE
0	No response
1+	Sluggish or diminished
2+	Active or expected response
3+	More brisk than expected, slightly hyperactive
4+	Brisk, hyperactive, with intermittent or transient clonus

TECHNIQUE

FINDINGS

■ *Triceps*
Flex patient's arm at elbow up to 90 degrees and rest patient's hand against the side of the body. Palpate triceps tendon and strike directly with reflex hammer, just above elbow.

EXPECTED: Visible or palpable extension of elbow, contraction of triceps muscle.

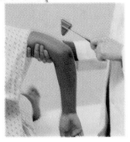

■ *Patellar*
Flex patient's knee up to 90 degrees, allowing lower leg to hang loosely. Support upper leg so it does not rest against edge of examining table, then strike patellar tendon just below patella.

EXPECTED: Extension of lower leg, contraction of quadriceps muscle.

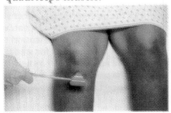

TECHNIQUE   FINDINGS

■ *Achilles*
Ask patient to sit. Then
flex patient's knee and
dorsiflex ankle up to 90
degrees, holding heel of
foot. Strike Achilles tendon at level of ankle
malleoli.

EXPECTED: Plantar flexion,
contraction of gastrocnemius
muscle.

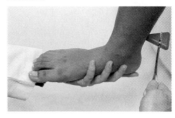

■ *Clonus*
Support patient's knee in
partially flexed position
and briskly dorsiflex the
foot with other hand,
maintaining foot in
flexion.

UNEXPECTED: Sustained
clonus, rhythmic oscillating
movements between dorsiflexion and plantar flexion
palpated.

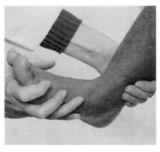

AIDS TO DIFFERENTIAL DIAGNOSIS

ABNORMALITY	DESCRIPTION
Generalized seizure disorder	Episodic, sudden, involuntary contractions of a group of muscles. Disturbances in conscious behavior, sensation, autonomic functioning, and urinary and fecal incontinence may accompany seizures.
Meningitis	Fever, chills, nuchal rigidity, headache, seizures, and vomiting, followed by alterations in level of consciousness. ***Can be life threatening.***
Encephalitis	Inflammation of brain and spinal cord that often begins as a mild, febrile viral illness, often followed by a quiescent stage. Then central nervous system (CNS) disturbances such as headache, drowsiness, and confusion, lead to stupor and coma. Possible motor function impairment with severe paralysis or ataxia.
Lesions (intracranial)	Headaches, vomiting, change in cognition, motor dysfunction, seizures, and personality changes.
Cerebrovascular accident (stroke)	Sudden, focal neurologic deficit with signs of restlessness, lethargy, changes in level of consciousness, vital sign and pupil changes, and impaired communication.

ABNORMALITY	DESCRIPTION
Parkinson disease	Initial symptoms: tremors at rest and with fatigue that disappear with movement and sleep. Progression tremor of head; slowing of voluntary movement; bilateral pill-rolling of fingers; delays in execution of movement; masked facial expression; poor blink rate; short, shuffling steps; slowed, slurred, and monotonous speech; and possible behavioral changes and dementia.
Peripheral neuropathy	Decreased or loss of pain, vibratory, and temperature sensation; absent reflexes and muscle wasting in affected extremity sometimes occurs.
Cerebral palsy	Alterations in muscle tone, posture, motor performance, and reflexes.

Clinical Signs of Motor Neuron Lesions

UPPER MOTOR NEURON	LOWER MOTOR NEURON
Muscle spasticity, possible contractures	Muscle flaccidity
Little or no muscle atrophy, but decreased strength	Loss of muscle tone and strength; muscle atrophy
Hyperactive deep tendon and abdominal reflexes; absent plantar reflex	Weak or absent deep tendon, plantar, and abdominal reflexes
No fasciculations	Fasciculations
Damage above level of brainstem will affect opposite side of body	Changes in muscles supplied by that nerve, usually a muscle on same side as the lesion
Paralysis of lower part of face, if involved	Bell palsy, if face involved; coordination unimpaired

PEDIATRIC VARIATIONS

EXAMINATION

Neurologic findings in the infant and child change as the child matures. For a complete description of anticipated maturational findings see Chapter 20.

TECHNIQUE	FINDINGS

Indirectly evaluate cranial nerve in newborns and infants

- *Optical blink reflex (CN II, III, IV)*
  Shine a light at the infant's open eyes. Observe the quick closure of the eyes and dorsal flexion of the infant's head.

  EXPECTED: Gazes intensely at close object or face. Focuses on and tracks an object with both eyes.
  UNEXPECTED: No response may indicate poor light perception.

- *Rooting reflex (CN V)*
  Touch one corner of the infant's mouth. The infant should open its mouth and turn its head in the direction of stimulation.

  EXPECTED: If infant has been recently fed, minimal or no response is expected.

- *Sucking reflex (CN V)*
  Place your finger in the infant's mouth, feeling the sucking action. Note the pressure, strength, and pattern of sucking.

  EXPECTED: The tongue should push up against your finger with good strength.

- *Infant's facial expression (CN VII)*
  Observe and note the infant's ability to wrinkle the forehead when crying and the symmetry of the smile.

  EXPECTED: Facial symmetry with all expressions.

TECHNIQUE	FINDINGS
■ *Acoustic blink reflex (CN VIII)* Loudly clap your hands about 30 cm from the infant's head; avoid producing an air current. Note the blink in response to the sound.	**EXPECTED:** Infant will habituate to repeated testing. Moves eyes in direction of sound. Freezes position with high-pitched sound. **UNEXPECTED:** No response after 2 to 3 days of age may indicate hearing problems.
■ *Doll's eye maneuver (CN VIII)* Hold the infant under the axilla in an upright position, head held steady, facing you. Rotate the infant first in one direction and then in the other.	**EXPECTED:** The infant's eyes should turn in the direction of rotation and then the opposite direction when rotation stops. **UNEXPECTED:** If the eyes do not move in the expected direction, suspect a vestibular problem or eye muscle paralysis.
■ *Swallowing and gag reflex (CN IX and X)* ■ *Coordinated sucking and swallowing ability (CN XII)* Pinch infant's nose.	**EXPECTED:** Mouth will open and tip of tongue will rise in a midline position.

Evaluate primitive reflexes in infant

■ *Palmar grasp (present at birth)* Making sure the infant's head is in midline, touch the palm of the infant's hand from the ulnar side (opposite the thumb). Note the strong grasp of your finger. Sucking facilitates the grasp.	**EXPECTED:** Grasp should be strongest between 1 and 2 months of age and disappear by 3 months.

TECHNIQUE	FINDINGS
■ *Plantar grasp (present at birth)* Touch the plantar surface of the infant's feet at the base of the toes.	**EXPECTED:** The toes should curl downward. The reflex should be strong up to 8 months of age.
■ *Moro reflex (present at birth)* With the infant supported in semisitting position, allow the head and trunk to drop back to a 30-degree angle. Observe symmetric abduction and extension of the arms.	**EXPECTED:** Fingers fan out and thumb and index finger form a C. The arms then adduct in an embracing motion followed by relaxed flexion. The reflex diminishes in strength by 3 to 4 months and disappears by 6 months.
■ *Placing (4 days of age)* Hold the infant upright under the arms next to a table or chair. Touch the dorsal side of the foot to the table or chair edge.	**EXPECTED:** Observe flexion of the hips and knees and lifting of the foot as if stepping up on the table. Age of disappearance varies.
■ *Stepping (between birth and 8 weeks)* Hold the infant upright under the arms and allow the soles of the feet to touch the surface of the table.	**EXPECTED:** Observe for alternate flexion and extension of the legs, simulating walking. It disappears before voluntary walking.
■ Asymmetric *tonic neck or "fencing" (by 2 to 3 months)* With the infant lying supine and relaxed or sleeping, turn its head to one side so the jaw is over the shoulder.	**EXPECTED:** Observe for extension of the arm and leg on the side to which the head is turned and for flexion of the opposite arm and leg.
Turn the infant's head to the other side.	**EXPECTED:** Observe the reversal of the extremities' posture. This reflex diminishes at 3 to 4 months of age and disappears by 6 months.

TECHNIQUE	FINDINGS
	UNEXPECTED: Be concerned if the infant never exhibits the reflex or seems locked in the fencing position.

Evaluate Neurologic Soft Signs in Children

(Age [in years] at which finding becomes unexpected noted in parentheses.)

■ *Walking, running gait*	**UNEXPECTED:** Stiff-legged with a foot slapping quality, unusual posturing of the arm (3).
■ *Heel walking*	**UNEXPECTED:** Difficulty remaining on heels for a distance of 10 ft (7).
■ *Tip-toe walking*	**UNEXPECTED:** Difficulty remaining on toes for a distance of 10 ft (7).
■ *Tandem gait*	**UNEXPECTED:** Difficulty walking heel-to-toe, unusual posturing of arms (7).
■ *One-foot standing*	**UNEXPECTED:** Unable to remain standing on one foot longer than 5 to 10 sec (5).
■ *Hopping in place*	**UNEXPECTED:** Unable to rhythmically hop on each foot (6).
■ *Motor-stance*	**UNEXPECTED:** Difficulty maintaining stance (arms extended in front, feet together, and eyes closed), drifting of arms, mild writhing movements of hands or fingers (3).
■ *Visual tracking*	**UNEXPECTED:** Difficulty following object with eyes when keeping the head still; nystagmus (5).
■ *Rapid thumb-to-finger test*	**UNEXPECTED:** Rapid touching thumb to fingers in sequence is uncoordinated; unable to suppress mirror movements in contralateral hand (8).

TECHNIQUE	FINDINGS
■ *Rapid alternating movements of hands*	**UNEXPECTED:** Irregular speed and rhythm with pronation and supination of hands patting the knees (10).
■ *Finger-nose test*	**UNEXPECTED:** Unable to alternately touch examiner's finger and own nose consecutively (7).
■ *Right-left discrimination*	**UNEXPECTED:** Unable to identify right and left sides of own body (5).
■ *Two-point discrimination*	**UNEXPECTED:** Difficulty in localizing and discriminating when touched in one or two places (6).
■ *Graphesthesia*	**UNEXPECTED:** Unable to identify geometric shapes you draw in child's open hand (8).
■ *Stereognosis*	**UNEXPECTED:** Unable to identify common objects placed in own hand (5).

Modified from Smith and McNamara, 1984.

SAMPLE DOCUMENTATION

Cranial nerves I-XII. Grossly intact.

Proprioception and cerebellar function. Gait is coordinated and even. Romberg negative. Rapid alternating movements coordinated and smooth.

Sensory function. Superficial touch, pain, and vibratory sensation intact bilaterally.

Reflexes. Deep tendon reflex 2+ bilaterally in all extremities. Plantar reflex produces expected plantar flexion of toes; no ankle clonus.

CHAPTER 18

HEAD-TO-TOE EXAMINATION: ADULT

COMPONENTS OF THE EXAMINATION

Because there is no one correct way to order the parts of the physical examination, you are encouraged to consider the following suggested approach for a particular setting, patient condition, or patient disability.

General Inspection

Start the examination when the patient is within your view. As you first observe the patient, take note of the following:

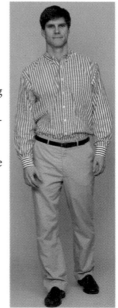

Signs of distress or disease
Habitus
Manner of sitting
Degree of relaxation on the face
Relationship with others in the room
Degree of interest in what is happening
    in the room

On greeting the patient, assess the following:

Alacrity with which you are met
Moistness of the palm when you shake
    hands
Eyes: luster and expression of emotion
Skin color
Facial expression
Mobility:
    Use of assistive devices
    Gait
    Sitting, rising from chair
    Taking off coat
Dress and posture

Speech pattern, disorders, foreign language
Difficulty hearing, assistive devices
Stature and build
Musculoskeletal deformities
Vision problems, assistive devices
Eye contact with you
Orientation, mental alertness
Nutritional state
Respiratory problems
Significant others accompanying patient

Patient Instructions

Empty the bladder.
Remove as much clothing as is necessary.
Put on a gown.

Measurements

Measure height.
Measure weight.
Assess distance vision: Snellen chart.
Document vital signs: temperature, pulse, respiration, blood pressure in both arms.

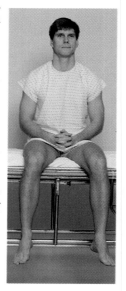

Patient Seated, Wearing Gown

Stand in front of patient seated on examining table.

Head and face

Inspect skin characteristics.
Inspect symmetry and external characteristics of eyes and ears.
Inspect configuration of skull.
Inspect and palpate scalp and hair for texture, distribution, and quantity of hair.
Palpate facial bones.
Palpate temporomandibular joint while patient opens and closes mouth.

Palapte sinus regions; if tender, transilluminate.

Inspect ability to clench teeth, squeeze eyes tightly shut, wrinkle forehead, smile, stick out tongue, puff out cheeks (CN V, VII).

Test light sensation of forehead, cheeks, chin (CN V).

Eyes

External examination.

Inspect eyelids, eyelashes, palpebral folds.

Determine alignment of eyebrows.

Inspect sclerae, conjunctivae, irides.

Palpate lacrimal apparatus.

Near-vision screening: Rosenbaum chart (CN II).

Eye function:

Test pupillary response to light and accommodation.

Perform cover-uncover test and light reflex.

Test extraocular eye movements (CN III, IV, VI).

Assess visual fields (CN II).

Test corneal reflexes (CN V).

Ophthalmoscopic examination:

Test red reflex

Inspect lens.

Inspect disc, cup margins, vessels, retinal surface, vitreous humor.

Ears

Inspect alignment.

Inspect surface characteristics.

Palpate auricle.

Assess hearing with whisper test or ticking watch (CN VIII).

Perform otoscopic examination:

Inspect canals.

Inspect tympanic membranes for landmarks, deformities, inflammation

Use a tuning fork to assess bone and air conduction.

Nose

Note structure, position of septum.

Determine patency of each nostril.

Inspect mucosa, septum, and turbinates with nasal speculum.

Assess olfactory function when indicated: test sense of smell (CN I).

Mouth and pharynx

Inspect lips, buccal mucosa, gums, hard and soft palates, floor of mouth for color and surface characteristics.

Inspect oropharynx: note anteroposterior pillars, uvula, tonsils, posterior pharynx, mouth odor.

Inspect teeth for color, number, surface characteristics.

Inspect tongue for color, characteristics, symmetry, movement (CN XII).

Test gag reflex and "ah" reflex (CN IX, X).

Perform sense of taste test (CN VII and IX) when indicated.

Neck

Inspect for symmetry and smoothness of neck and thyroid.

Inspect for jugular venous distention.

Perform active and passive range of motion; test resistance against examiner's hand.

Test strength of shoulder shrug (CN XI).

Palpate carotid pulses. Be sure to palpate one side at a time.

Palpate tracheal position.

Palpate thyroid.

Palpate lymph nodes: preauricular and postauricular, occipital, tonsillar, submental, submandibular, superficial cervical chain, posterior cervical, deep cervical, supraclavicular.

Auscultate carotid arteries and thyroid.

Upper extremities

Observe and palpate hands, arms, and shoulders.

Skin and nail characteristics

Muscle mass

Muscular strength

Musculoskeletal deformities

Joint range of motion: fingers, wrists, elbows, shoulders

Assess pulses: radial, brachial.

Palpate epitrochlear nodes.

Patient Seated, Back Exposed

Stand behind patient seated on examining table.

Have males pull gown down to the waist so the entire chest and back are exposed.

Have females expose back; keep breasts covered.

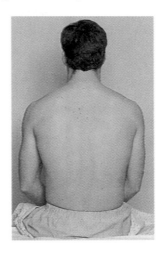

Back and posterior chest

Inspect skin and thoracic configuration.

Inspect symmetry of shoulders, musculoskeletal development.

Inspect and palpate scapulae and spine.

Palpate and percuss costovertebral angle.

Lungs

Inspect respiration: excursion, depth, rhythm, pattern.

Palpate for expansion and tactile fremitus.

Palpate scapular and subscapular nodes.

Percuss posterior chest and lateral walls systematically for resonance.

Percuss for diaphragmatic excursion.

Auscultate systematically for breath sounds (egophony, bronchophony, and whispered pectoriloquy): note characteristics and adventitious sounds.

Patient Seated, Chest Exposed

Move around to the front of the patient.
Have females lower gown to expose the anterior chest.

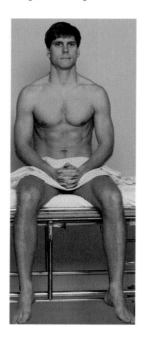

Anterior chest, lungs, and heart

Inspect skin, musculoskeletal development, symmetry.
Inspect respirations: patient posture, respiratory effort.
Inspect for pulsations or heaving.
Palpate chest wall for stability, crepitation, tenderness.
Palpate precordium for thrills, heaves, pulsations.
Palpate left chest to locate apical impulse.
Palpate for tactile fremitus.
Palpate nodes: infraclavicular, axillary.
Percuss systematically for breath sounds.
Auscultate systematically for heart sounds: aortic area, pulmonic area, second pulmonic area, tricuspid area, mitral area.

Female breasts

Inspect in these positions: patient's arms extended over head, pushing hands on hips, hands pushed together in front of chest, patient leaning forward.

Palpate breasts in all four quadrants, tail of Spence, over areolae; if breasts are large, perform bimanual palpation.

Palpate nipple: compress to observe for discharge.

Male breasts

Inspect breasts and nipples for symmetry, enlargement, surface characteristics.

Palpate breast tissue.

Patient Reclining 45 Degrees

Assist the patient to a reclining position at a 45-degree angle.

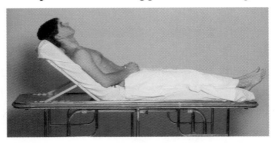

Stand to the side of the patient that allows the greatest comfort.

Inspect chest in recumbent position.

Inspect jugular venous pulsations and measure jugular venous pressure.

Patient Supine, Chest Exposed

Assist the patient into a supine position.

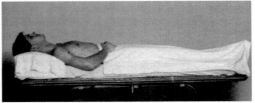

If the patient cannot tolerate lying flat, maintain head elevation at a 30-degree angle.

Uncover the chest while keeping the abdomen and lower extremities draped.

Female breasts

Inspect in recumbent position.

Palpate systematically with the patient's arm over her head and with her arm at her side.

Heart

Palpate the chest wall for thrills, heaves, pulsations.

Auscultate systematically; turn the patient slightly to the left side and repeat auscultation.

Patient Supine, Abdomen Exposed

Have the patient remain supine.

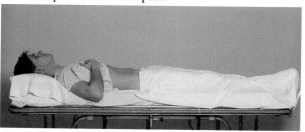

Cover the chest with the patient's gown.

Arrange draping to expose the abdomen from pubis to epigastrium.

Abdomen

Inspect skin characteristics, contour, pulsations, movement.

Auscultate all quadrants for bowel sounds.

Auscultate the aorta, renal arteries, and femoral arteries for bruits or venous hums.

Percuss all quadrants for tone.

Percuss liver borders and estimate span.

Percuss left midaxillary line for splenic dullness.

Lightly palpate all quadrants.

Deeply palpate all quadrants.

ID
age, sex, DOB

CC
reason for seeking care

HPI
O-onset
L-location
D-duration
C-character
A-aggravating/associated factors
R-relieving factors
T-temporal factors
S-severity
medications, treatments

PMH
general health, surgeries, hospitalizations, illnesses, immunizations, medications, allergies, blood transfusions, emotional status/psychiatric history

PERSONAL HISTORY
cultural background, marital status, occupation, economic resources, environment

HEALTH HABITS
tobacco; alcohol; illicit drugs; life-style, diet, exercise; exposure to toxins

HEALTH MAINTENANCE
last PE; diagnostic tests-date, result, follow-up; self-exams-breast, genital, testicular; last Pap smear, mammogram

FAMILY HISTORY
(parents, siblings, children) cancer, DM, hypertension, heart disease, stroke

GENERAL
fever, chills, malaise, fatigue/energy, night sweats; desired weight

DIET
appetite, restrictions, vitamins, supplements

SKIN, HAIR, NAILS
rash, eruptions, itching, pigment changes

HEAD & NECK
headaches, dizziness, head injuries, loss of consciousness

EYES
blurring, double vision, visual changes, glasses, trauma, eye diseases

EARS
hearing loss, pain, discharge, vertigo, tinnitus

NOSE
congestion, nose bleeds, postnasal drip

THROAT & MOUTH
hoarseness, sore throat, bleeding gums, ulcers, tooth problems

GASTROINTESTINAL
indigestion, heartburn, vomiting, bowel regularity/changes

LYMPH
tenderness, enlargement

ENDOCRINE
heat/cold intolerance, weight change, polydipsia, polyuria, hair changes; increased hat, glove or shoe size

FEMALE
LMP, age @ menarche; gravity, parity; menses-onset, regularity, duration, symptoms, sexual life (# partners, satisfaction), contraception, menopause (age, symptoms)

MALE
puberty onset, erections, testicular pain, libido, infertility

BREASTS
pain, tenderness, lumps, discharge

CHEST & LUNGS
cough, sputum, shortness of breath, dyspnea on exertion, night sweats; exposure to TB

CARDIOVASCULAR
chest pain, palpations, number of pillows, edema, claudication, exercise tolerance

HEMATOLOGY
anemia, easy bruising

GENITOURINARY
dysuria, flank pain, urgency, frequency, nocturia, hematuria, dribbling

MUSCULOSKELETAL
joint pain, heat swelling

NEUROLOGIC
fainting, weakness, loss of coordination

MENTAL STATUS
concentration, sleeping, eating, socialization, mood changes, suicidal thoughts

VS
TPR, BP, Ht, Wt

GENERAL APPEARANCE
age, race, gender, posture and gait

MENTAL STATUS
consciousness, cognitive ability, memory, emotional stability, thought content, speech quality

SKIN
color, integrity, hygiene, turgor, hydration, edema, lesions; hair distribution, texture; nail texture, nail base angle

HEAD
scalp; temporal arteries; deformities

NECK
trachea (position, tug) range of motion (ROM); carotid bruit; jugular venous distention (JVD); thyroid; lymph-head & neck

EYES
pupils (PERRLA) eyelids, conjunctivae, sclerae, EOMs (CN III, IV, VI), light reflex, visual fields, funduscopy (CN II); acuity (CN II), nystagmus

EARS
deformities, lesions, discharge, otoscopy (canal, TM), hearing (Rinne, Weber; CN VIII)

NOSE
mucosa, septum, turbinates, discharge, sinus area swelling or tenderness

MOUTH & THROAT
lips/teeth/gums, tongue (CN XII), mucosa, palates, tonsils, exudate, uvula, gag reflex (CN IX, X)

CHEST/LUNGS
shape, movement, respirations (rate, rhythm); expansion, accessory muscles, tactile fremitus, crepitus, percussion tone, excursion, auscultation (clear, wheeze, crackles, rhonchi, rubs)

BREASTS
contour, symmetry, nipples, areolae, discharge, lumps/masses; lymph-axillary, supraclavicular & infraclavicular

HEART
PMI, lifts, thrills, rate, rhythm, S1, S2, splitting, gallops, rubs, murmurs, snaps

BLOOD VESSELS
cyanosis, clubbing, edema; peripheral pulses, skin, nails

ABDOMEN
contour, symmetry, skin, bowel sounds, bruits, hum, liver span, liver border, tenderness, masses, spleen, kidneys, aortic pulsation; reflexes, percussion tone; costovertebral angle (CVA) tenderness; femoral pulses; lymph-inguinal

MALE GENITALIA
pubic hair, glans, penis, testis, scrotum, epididymis, urethral discharge, hernias

FEMALE GENITALIA
external lesions or discharge, Bartholin and Skene glands, urethra, vaginal walls, cervix (position, lesions, cervical motion tenderness), uterus, adnexae

RECTUM/PROSTATE
sacrococcygeal & perianal areas, anus, sphincter tone, rectal walls, masses, fecal occult blood test (FOBT),
<u>Male</u>-prostate
<u>Female</u>-rectovaginal septum, uterus

MUSCULOSKELETAL
posture, alignment, symmetry, joint heat/swelling/color; muscle tone; ROM; strength

NEUROLOGIC
CN II-XII, rapid alternating movements, finger to nose; sensation; vibration; stereognosis; motor system, gait Romberg; deep tendon reflexes (DTRs); superficial reflexes

Cranial Nerves
I-smell
II-visual acuity; visual fields, funduscopy
III, IV, VI-eyelid opening EOMs: IV up and out; VI lateral; III all others
V-corneal reflex, facial sensation (3 areas); jaw opening, bite strength
VII-eyebrow raise, eyelid close, smile, taste
VIII-Rinne, Weber
IX, X-gag reflex, palate elevation, phonation
XI-lateral head rotation, neck flexion, shoulder shrug
XII-tongue protrusion; lateral deviation strength

Palpate right costal margin for liver border.

Palpate left costal margin for spleen.

Palpate for right and left kidneys.

Palpate midline for aortic pulsation.

Test abdominal reflexes.

Have patient raise the head as you inspect the abdominal muscles.

Inguinal area

Palpate for lymph nodes, pulses, hernias.

External genitalia, males

Inspect penis, urethral meatus, scrotum, pubic hair.

Palpate scrotal contents (you may want to have the patient assume an alternate position, such as standing or sitting).

Patient Supine, Legs Exposed

Have patient remain supine.

Arrange drapes to cover the abdomen and pubis and to expose the lower extremities.

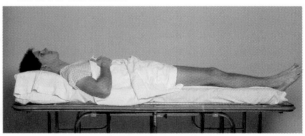

Feet and legs

Inspect for skin characteristics, hair distribution, muscle mass, musculoskeletal configuration.

Palpate for temperature, texture, edema, pulses (dorsalis pedis, posterior tibial, popliteal).

Test range of motion and strength of toes, feet, ankles, knees.

Hips

Palpate hips for stability.

Test range of motion and strength of hips.

Patient Sitting, Lap Draped

Assist the patient to a sitting position.
Have patient wear gown with a drape across the lap.

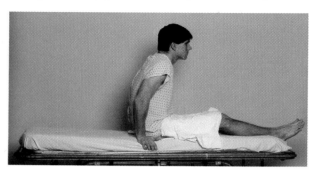

Musculoskeletal

Observe patient moving from lying to sitting position.
Note coordination, use of muscles, muscle strength, ease of movement.

Neurologic

Test sensory function: dull and sharp sensation of forehead, cheeks, chin, lower arms, hands, lower legs, feet.
Test vibratory sensation of wrists, ankles.
Test two-point discrimination of palms, thighs, back.
Test stereognosis, graphesthesia.
Test fine motor function, coordination, and position sense of upper extremities, asking patient to:
  Touch nose with alternating index fingers.
  Rapidly alternate touching fingers to thumb.
  Rapidly move index finger between own nose and examiner's finger.
Test fine motor function, coordination, and position sense of lower extremities, asking patient to:
  Run heel down tibia of opposite leg.
  Alternately and rapidly cross leg over opposite knee.
Test deep tendon reflexes and compare bilaterally: biceps, triceps, brachioradial, patellar, Achilles.
Test the plantar reflex bilaterally.

Patient Standing

Assist patient to a standing position.
Stand next to patient.

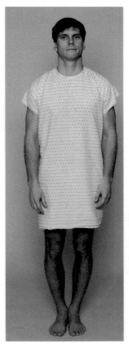

Spine

Inspect and palpate spine as patient bends over at waist.
Test range of motion: hyperextension, lateral bending, rotation
of upper trunk.

Neurologic

Observe gait.
Test proprioception and cerebellar function:
Perform Romberg test
Ask the patient to walk heel to toe.
Ask the patient to stand on one foot, then the other, with
eyes closed.

Ask the patient to hop in place on one foot, then the other.
Ask the patient to do deep knee bends.

Abdominal/genital

Test for inguinal and femoral hernias.

Female Patient, Lithotomy Position

Assist female patient into lithotomy position, and drape appropriately.
Sit next to patient.

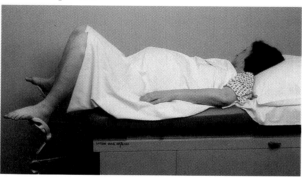

External genitalia

Inspect pubic hair, labia, clitoris, urethral opening, vaginal opening, perineal and perianal area, anus.
Palpate labia and Bartholin glands; milk Skene glands.

Internal genitalia

Perform speculum examination:
    Inspect vagina and cervix.
    Collect Pap smear and other necessary specimens.
Perform bimanual palpation to assess for characteristics of vagina, cervix, uterus, adnexae.
Perform rectovaginal examination to assess rectovaginal septum, broad ligaments.
Perform rectal examination:
    Assess anal sphincter tone and surface characteristics.
    Obtain rectal culture if needed.
    Note characteristics of stool when gloved finger is removed.

Male Patient, Bending Forward

Assist male patient in leaning over examining table or into knee-chest position. Stand behind patient.

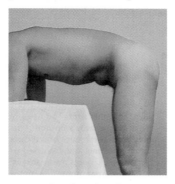

Inspect sacrococcygeal and perianal areas.
Perform rectal examination:
    Palpate sphincter tone and surface characteristics.
    Obtain rectal culture if needed.
    Palpate prostate gland and seminal vesicles.
    Note characteristics of stool when gloved finger is removed.

Examination Conclusion

Allow patient to dress in private.
Share findings and interpretations with patient.
Answer any of the patient's additional questions.
Confirm that the patient has a clear understanding of all aspects of the situation.
If the patient is examined in a hospital bed:
    Put everything back in order when finished.
    Make sure the patient is comfortably settled in an appropriate manner.
    Put bed side rails up if the clinical condition warrants it.
    Make sure that buttons and buzzers are within easy reach.

CLINICAL AND
REFERENCE NOTES

CHAPTER 19

THE HEALTHY FEMALE EVALUATION

The following are items to consider for inclusion as part of a routine well-woman visit. This is not intended as an all-inclusive list. Some items may vary depending upon the woman's age, health status, and particular risk factors. Past medical history (PMH) and review of systems (ROS) may also be appropriate if indicated. Age and risk-status guidelines for preventive services are available from a variety of sources and authorities.*

HISTORY

History of Present Illness (HPI)

Age
Last normal menstrual period (LNMP)
Menopause: age achieved, symptoms
Obstetric history: number of pregnancies, term pregnancies, preterm pregnancies, abortions/miscarriages, and living children (GPTAL)
Contraceptive measures and history
Sexual history
Unusual vaginal bleeding or discharge
Abdominal or pelvic pain
Urinary symptoms

U.S. Preventive Services Task Force, *Guide to Clinical Preventive Services,* ed. 2, 1996; U.S. D.H.H.S., *Clinician's Handbook of Preventive Services,* 1994.
Authorities that produce prevention guidelines include Academy of Family Physicians, American Cancer Society, American College of Obstetricians and Gynecologists, American College of Physicians, American Geriatrics Society, Canadian Task Force on the Periodic Health Examination, National Cancer Institute, and U.S. Preventive Services Task Force.

Risk Assessment

Cardiovascular: smoking, hypertension, diet, weight, exercise, family history

Cancer: personal/family history of breast, ovarian cancer

Infection: Sexually transmitted disease (STD) exposure

Metabolic: calcium supplement; family history of osteoporosis; exercise; personal/family history of diabetes mellitus

Injury: alcohol, seat belts, guns, family violence

Depression: vegetative symptoms (eating, sleeping, concentration, energy, social interaction)

Health Habits

Breast self-examination

Pap smear: how often; date of last pap smear; results; ever have an abnormal result

Mammogram: date of last mammogram; results

Diet: fat, cholesterol, calcium

Exercise

Smoking

Alcohol/drugs

PHYSICAL EXAMINATION

Vital signs

Height and weight; body mass index (BMI)

Skin: lesions, moles

Lungs

Cardiovascular and peripheral vascular

Breasts: contour, masses; nipple discharge

Lymph: regional lymphadenopathy (infraclavicular and supraclavicular, axillary)

Pelvic: lesions, discharge; Bartholin glands, urethra, Skene glands; vagina, cervix, adnexa, uterus

Rectal: hemorrhoids, masses, lesions

SCREENING TESTS

Pap smear: frequency depends on age, sexual status, PMH, past Pap smear history

STD testing: depending on exposure status

Mammogram: frequency depends on age, personal and family history, past results

Fecal occult blood test: depending on age, personal and family history

Cholesterol/lipid profile: depending on age, personal and family history

CLINICAL AND
REFERENCE NOTES

CHAPTER 20

HEAD-TO-TOE EXAMINATION: INFANTS, CHILDREN, AND ADOLESCENTS

EXAMINATION GUIDELINES

The approach to a pediatric physical examination must, of course, be age appropriate. Not every observation must be made in every child at every examination. What you do depends on the individual circumstance and on your clinical judgment. Each step must be considered in relation to the patient's age, physical condition, and emotional state. The order of the examination can be modified according to need; it should not be stereotypical. Care should be given to assure the safety of the child on the examining table. During the pre-elementary school years (and sometimes later), an adult's lap is often a better site for much and often all of the examination.

Your notes should include a description of the child's behavior during interactions with the parent (or a surrogate) and with you.

Take the child's temperature, weight, and length or height. Take the blood pressure and record the extremity (ies), size of cuff, and method used.

Note percentiles for all measurements.

Depending upon clinical requirements, consider including arm span, upper segment measurement (crown to top of symphysis), lower segment measurement (symphysis to soles of feet), upper/lower segment ratio, and head and chest circumference.

Offer toys or paper and pencil to entertain the child (if age appropriate), to develop rapport, and to evaluate development, motor and neurologic status.

Use a developmental screening test such as the Denver II to evaluate language, motor coordination, and social skills.

Evaluate mental status as the child interacts with you and with the parent.

Take advantage of opportunities the child presents during the examination to make your observations.

Child Playing

While the child plays on the floor, evaluate the musculoskeletal and neurologic systems while developing a rapport with the child.

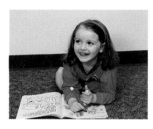

Observe the child's spontaneous activities.

Ask the child to demonstrate skills such as throwing a ball, building block towers, drawing geometric figures, coloring.

Evaluate gait, jumping, hopping, range of motion.

Muscle strength: Observe the child climbing on the parent's lap, stooping and recovering.

Child on Parent's Lap

Perform the examination on the parent's lap to enhance the child's participation.

Begin with the child sitting and undressed except for the diaper or underpants.

Upper extremities

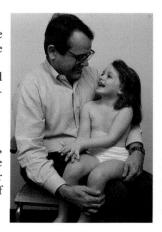

Inspect arms for movement, size, shape; observe use of the hands; inspect hands for number and configuration of fingers, palmar creases.

Palpate radial pulses.

Elicit biceps and triceps reflexes when child cooperates.

Take blood pressure at this point or later, depending on child's attitude.

Lower extremities

Child may stand for much or part of the examination.

Inspect legs for movement, size, shape, alignment, lesions.

Inspect feet for alignment, longitudinal arch, number of toes.

Palpate femoral and dorsalis pedis pulses.

Elicit plantar reflex and, if child is cooperative, the Achilles and patellar reflexes.

Head and neck

Inspect head.

Inspect shape, alignment with neck, hairline, position of auricles.

Palpate anterior fontanel for size; head for sutures, depressions; hair for texture.

Measure head circumference.

Inspect neck for webbing, voluntary movement.

Palpate neck: position of trachea, thyroid, muscle tone, lymph nodes.

Chest, heart, and lungs

Inspect the chest for respiratory movement, size, shape, precordial movement, deformity, nipple and breast development.

Palpate the anterior chest, locate the point of maximal impulse, note tactile fremitus in the talking or crying child.

Auscultate the anterior, lateral, and posterior chest for breath sounds; count respirations.

Auscultate all cardiac listening areas for S_1 and S_2, splitting, and murmurs; count apical pulse.

Child Relatively Supine, Still on Lap, Diaper Loosened

Inspect abdomen.

Auscultate for bowel sounds.

Palpate: Identify size of the liver and any other palpable organs or masses.

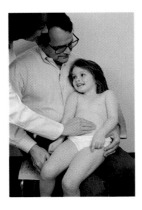

Percuss.

Palpate the femoral pulses, compare to radial pulses.

Palpate for lymph nodes.

Inspect the external genitalia.

Males: Palpate scrotum for descent of testes and other masses.

Child Standing

Inspect spinal alignment as the child bends slowly forward to touch toes.

Observe posture from anterior, posterior, and lateral views.

Observe gait.

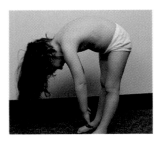

Child on Parent's Lap

Prepare child for examination

Only if absolutely necessary, restrain the child for funduscopic, otoscopic, and oral examinations.

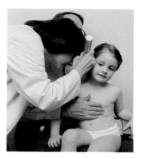

Lessen the fear of these examinations by permitting the child to handle the instruments, blow out the light, or use them on a doll or on the parent.

Attempt to gain the child's cooperation, even if it takes more time; future visits will be more pleasant for both of you.

After finishing these preliminary maneuvers, perform the following:

> Inspect eyes: corneal light reflex, red reflex, extraocular movements, funduscopic examination.
>
> Perform otoscopic examination. Note the position and description of the pinnae.
>
> Inspect nasal mucosa.
>
> Inspect mouth and pharynx. Note the numbers of teeth, deciduous or permanent, and any special characteristics.

(NOTE: By the time the child is of school age, it is usually possible to use an examination sequence very similar to that for adults.) See pp. 296-303 for examples of forms used to chart physical growth.

AGE-SPECIFIC ANTICIPATED OBSERVATIONS AND GUIDELINES*

Keep in mind that this is a suggested outline, always modified by human variation, and that all percentages are subject to gaussian distribution. History taking can be facilitated by referring to baby

---

*Adapted from clinic forms used in the Primary Care Continuity Clinic in the Children's Medical Center at The Johns Hopkins Hospital under the leadership of Drs. Janet Servint and Kevin Johnson and from the pediatric section, authored by Henry M. Seidel, of "Clinical History and Physical Examination," a booklet prepared for second-year medical students at The Johns Hopkins School of Medicine under the direction of Lawrence S.C. Griffith, MD.

books, report cards, pictures, and other materials the family may have at home. Also, these suggestions assume a continuing relationship with the patient. Of course, you must begin with a full history and physical examination at whatever age you first see the patient.

2 Weeks of Age

History (particular attention)

Pertinent perinatal history
Social: sleeping arrangements, housing
Stool pattern
Umbilicus: healing, discharge, granulation
Diet: feeding modality, schedule

Development: By this age

80% will lift and turn head when in prone position
40% will follow an object to midline visually
35% will vocalize; become quiet in response to a voice
45% will regard a face intently, diminishing activity for the moment

Physical Examination (particular attention)

Establish growth curves (weight, height, head circumference)
Hips
Reflexes: Moro, root, grasp, step

Anticipatory Guidance (particular attention)

Sleep (emphasize supine position and avoidance of soft and fuzzy threats to safe breathing)
Feeding: use of pacifier (need to suck)
Use of bulb syringe (nasal stuffiness)
Safety: falling, crib sides, car seats
Skin care
Clothing
Illness: temperature taking
Crying (holding the baby)

Plans and Problems

What risks have revealed themselves as you got to know the family? What are apparent problems? Start a problem list and make appropriate dispositions
Consider the need for hemoglobin or hematocrit value

2 Months of Age

History (particular attention)

Expressions of parental concern
Child's apparent temperament
Sleep cycle
Feeding patterns, frequency
Stooling pattern, frequency, color, consistency, straining
Be certain there is no probability of immunocompromise in patient or relevant family members or other contacts (prior to starting immunizations)
Social issues:
  Father's involvement
  Living conditions
  Smokers, other concerning habits
  Any apparent high-risk concerns

Development: By this age

Gross motor:
  80% will lift head to 45 degrees in prone position
  45% will lift head to as much as 90 degrees in prone position
  25% will roll over stomach to back
Fine motor:
  99%+ will follow a moving object to the midline
  85% will follow a moving object past the midline
Language:
  Almost all will diminish activity at the sound of a voice
  35% will spontaneously vocalize
  Many will vocalize responsively
Psychosocial:
  Almost all will diminish activity when regarding a face
  Almost all will respond to a friendly, cooing face with a social smile
  50% may smile spontaneously or even laugh aloud

Physical Examination (particular attention)

Growth curves (weight, height, head circumference)
Hearing
Vision
Hips

Anticipatory Guidance

Feeding (delay or at least downplay solids, avoid citrus, wheat, mixed foods, eggs, minimize water)

When and if mother returns to work

Hiccups

Straining at stool

Visual and auditory stimulus (mobiles, mirrors, rattles, sing and talk to baby)

Sibling rivalry (if there are siblings)

Babysitters (checking references, assuring immunization status, reliability)

Safety (rolling over, playpen, car seat, discourage walker, no smoking)

Sleep (reemphasize location and supine position)

Smoking and its evils

Plans and Problems

Initiate immunizations and, throughout, attempt to follow American Academy of Pediatrics guidelines; at this visit and at every subsequent visit, discuss the benefits, risks, and side effects of immunizations (always remember the risks for the immunocompromised)

List problems, e.g., allergies, medications, any areas of concern, and make appropriate plans and, when necessary, referrals

Consider the need for hemoglobin or hematocrit value

4 Months of Age

History (particular attention)

Parental concerns

Infant's sleep cycle and temperament

Feeding patterns, frequency, mother's feelings if she is breast-feeding

Stooling pattern, frequency, color, consistency, straining

Social issues:

Father's involvement

Amplify early impressions of the home's social structure

Smokers, other concerning habits

Any apparent high-risk concerns

Development: By this age

Gross motor:

80%, when prone, will lift chest up with arm support

80% will roll over from stomach to back

35% will have no head lag when pulled to sitting position and many will then hold head steady when kept in that position

Fine motor:

60% will reach for a dangling object

Almost all will bring hands together

Almost all will follow a face or object up to 180 degrees

Language:

Almost all will laugh aloud

20% will appear to initiate vocalization

Psychosocial:

80% will smile spontaneously

Many will regard their own hand for several seconds

Physical Examination (particular attention)

Growth curves (weight, height, head circumference)

Reassess hearing

Reassess vision

Anticipatory Guidance

Introduction of solid food (cereal)

Stool changes with changes in diet

Drooling and teething

Thumb sucking, pacifiers, bottles at bedtime

Safety (aspiration, rolling over, holding baby with hot liquids, reemphasize earlier discussions, e.g., car seat)

Reemphasize environmental stimulus

Further discussion of babysitters

Use of antipyretics, e.g., acetaminophen

Plans and Problems

Review immunizations and implement as appropriate

Maintain problem list, making appropriate plans and, if necessary, referrals

Consider the need for a hematocrit or hemoglobin value

6 Months of Age

History (interim details)

Parental concerns
Sleep patterns
Diet
Stooling pattern
Further exploration of social issues
> If father has not attended these care visits regularly, encourage his participation (or if mother has not been consistent for whatever reason, address the relevant issues)

Development: By this age

Gross motor:
> 90%, pulled to a sitting position, will have no head lag
> 60% will sit alone
> 75% will bear some weight on legs
> Almost all will roll over

Fine motor:
> More than half will pass a toy from hand to hand
> 60%, in a sitting position, will look for a toy
> 40%, in a sitting position, will take two cubes

Language:
> 60% will turn toward a voice
> 30% will initiate speech sounds, e.g., ma-ma, da-da, but not specifically

Psychosocial:
> 30% may cry and turn away from strangers
> 40% may put an object in mouth to explore it, may feed self
> 60%, holding an object, may resist an attempt to pull it away

Physical Examination (particular attention)

Update growth curves
Double check on hearing and vision
Look for any possible new findings and recheck the old

Anticipatory Guidance

Bedtime routines (discuss putting child to bed while she is awake; waking up at night)
Fear of strangers
Separation anxiety

Safety (begin discussions about what toddlers can get into, cabinets, hot water, electrical outlets, medications and other poisons; inform about local poison control center, syrup of ipecac)

Shoes, when and if to use them

Teething, oral hygiene

Offering a cup

Checking fluoride intake

Addition of solid foods

Plans and Problems

Review immunizations and implement as appropriate

Consider the need for a serum lead level, hemoglobin or hematocrit value

Maintain problem list, making appropriate plans and, if necessary, referrals

9 Months of Age

History (interim details)

Parental concerns

Continued attention to sleep, diet, and stooling patterns

Continuing attention to social issues

Development: By this age

Gross motor:

Almost 100% will sit alone

80% will stand alone

45% will cruise

Some will have begun competent crawling

Fine motor:

70% will have thumb-finger grasp

60% will bang two cubes together

Almost all will finger feed

Language:

75% will imitate speech sounds

75% will use ma-ma, da-da nonspecifically

Psychosocial:

Almost 100% will try to get to a toy that is out of reach

85% will play repetitive games, e.g., peek-a-boo

45% will be shy with strangers and may cry

Physical Examination (particular attention)

Update growth curves

Constantly reassess earlier findings and look for anything new

Anticipatory Guidance

Oral hygiene, e.g., water without sugar in bottles (avoid tooth decay)

Sleep and the desirability of routine (naps, separation anxiety and how to deal with it)

Reemphasis on babysitters, references and reliability

Safety, e.g., stair gates and toddlers, falls, poisoning, burns, aspiration (never enough emphasis on safety, smoking, etc.)

Weaning, breast and/or bottle

Uses of discipline

Plans and Problems

Review immunizations and implement as appropriate

Consider the need for a serum lead level, hemoglobin, or hematocrit value

Maintain problem list, making appropriate plans and, if necessary, referrals

12 Months of Age

History (interim details)

Parental concerns

Reassess social and system review

Development: By this age

Gross motor:

85% will cruise

70% will stand alone briefly

50% will walk to some extent and more will try it with hands held

Fine motor:

90% will bang two cubes together

70% will have a good pincer grasp

Language:

80% will use ma-ma and da-da specifically

30% will use as many as three additional words

Almost all will indulge in immature jargoning

Psychosocial:

Almost all will respond to parent's presence and voice

Almost all will wave bye-bye

85% will play pat-a-cake

50% will drink from a cup

About half, perhaps a bit more, will play ball with examiner

Physical Examination (particular attention)

Update growth curves

Continued reassessment

Evaluate gait if walking has begun

Anticipatory Guidance

Many children this age begin to eat less; it is expected

Weaning (especially at night)

Increasing use of table food

Dental health, toothbrushing

Toilet training (expectations, attitudes)

Discipline, e.g., limit setting

Safety (child-proofing the house, street, lead paint, etc.)

Plans and Problems

Review immunizations and implement as appropriate

Consider the need for a serum lead level, hemoglobin or hematocrit value, tuberculosis test

Maintain problem list, making appropriate plans and, if necessary, referrals

15 Months of Age

History (interim details)

Parental concerns

Reassess social and system review

Development: By this age

Gross motor:

Almost all will walk well

Almost all will stoop to recover an object

35% will walk up steps with help

Fine motor:

Almost all will drink from a cup

Almost all will have a neat pincer grasp
70% will scribble with crayon
60% will make a tower with two cubes
Language:
Almost all will use ma-ma and da-da specifically
75% will use as many as three additional words
30% will put two words together
Psychosocial:
Many more than 50% will play ball with the examiner
50% will try to use a spoon
45% will try to remove clothing

Physical Examination (particular attention)

Update growth curves
Continued reassessment
Evaluate gait

Anticipatory Guidance

Negativism and independence
Dental health (visit to a dentist)
Toilet training
Weaning
Discipline, e.g., the need for consistency
Safety (all of the issues, repetitively)

Plans and Problems

Review immunizations and implement as appropriate
Consider the need for a serum lead level, hemoglobin or hematocrit value, tuberculosis test
Maintain problem list, making appropriate plans and, if necessary, referrals

18 Months of Age

History (interim details)

Parental concerns
Reassess social and system review

Development: By this age

Gross motor:

55% will have begun to walk up stairs without much help

70% will have started to walk backwards

More than that will have tried running with at least some success

45% will have tried with some success to kick a ball forward, given the opportunity

Fine motor:

80% will scribble if given a crayon

80% will make a tower with two cubes

About half of those will attempt with some success a tower of even as many as four cubes

Language:

Almost all will have mature jargoning

85% will have at least three words in addition to mama and dada

Many of those will put two words together

More than half will respond to a one-step command, e.g., when asked to point to a body part

Psychosocial

Well over half will assist with taking off their clothes

75% will use a spoon successfully, albeit with some spillage

Physical Examination (particular attention)

Update growth curves

Continued reassessment, search for new findings

Continue to evaluate gait

Anticipatory Guidance

Sleep (naps, nightmares)

Diet (mealtime battles)

Dental health (toothbrushing, dentist)

Toilet training

Discipline (methods and, again, consistency)

Safety (never enough discussion, e.g., seat belt, street and car, childproofing the home)

Self-comforting (masturbation, thumb sucking, favorite blankets and toys)

Child care settings if one is necessary

Plans and Problems

Review immunizations and implement as appropriate

Consider the need for serum lead level, hemoglobin or hematocrit value, tuberculosis test

Maintain problem list, making appropriate plans and, if necessary, referrals

2 Years of Age

History (interim details)

Parental concerns

Reassess social and system review

Development: By this age

Gross motor:

All should run well

All should walk up steps of reasonable height without holding on

90% will kick a ball forward

80% will throw a ball overhand

60% will do a little jump

40% may balance on one foot for 1 to 2 seconds

Fine motor:

Almost all should scribble with a pencil

90% will make a tower of 4 cubes

70% will copy a vertical line

Language:

All should point to and name parts of the body

85% will readily combine two different words

80% will understand "on" and "under"

75% will name a picture

Psychosocial:

85% will give a toy to mother or other significant person

60% will put on some clothing alone and, often, also remove a garment

50% will play games with others

Physical Examination (particular attention)

Update growth curves

Continued reassessment, search for new findings

Mouth and teeth; count the number of teeth

Anticipatory Guidance

Independence (limit setting, temper tantrums)
Peer interaction
Safety (poisons and potential poisons, water temperature, car safety seat use)
Toilet training
Nightmares
Use of a cup for drinking (as much as possible)

Plans and Problems

Review immunizations and implement as appropriate
Consider the need for serum lead level, hemoglobin or hematocrit value, dental referral, tuberculosis test
Maintain problem list, making appropriate plans and, if necessary, referrals

3 Years of Age

History (interim details)

Parental concerns
Reassess social and system review

Development: By this age

Gross motor:
75% will balance on one foot for at least one second
75% will negotiate a successful broad jump
40% will balance on one foot for as many as 5 seconds
Fine motor:
80% will copy a circle in addition to a vertical line
80% will build a tower of as many as 8 cubes
Language:
Speech is becoming more clearly understood in more than half
80% will use plurals appropriately
Almost half will give their first and last names appropriately
Psychosocial:
90% will put on clothing alone
75% will play interactive games
50% will separate from mother or other significant person without too much stress
Many will have begun to wash and dry hands

Physical Examination (particular attention)

Update growth curves
Continued reassessment, search for new findings
Are the teeth coming in appropriately

Anticipatory Guidance

Degrees of independence (limit setting and encouragement, a fine balance), other aspects of discipline
Safety (car seat, guns, strangers)
Personal hygiene (hand washing, toothbrushing, proper use of toilet tissue)
Day care

Plans and Problems

Review immunizations and implement as appropriate
Consider the need for serum lead level, hemoglobin or hematocrit value, tuberculosis test
Maintain problem list, making appropriate plans and, if necessary, referrals

4 Years of Age

History (interim details)

Parental concerns
Reassess social and system review

Development: By this age

Gross motor:
75% will hop on one foot
75% will balance on one foot for as many as 5 seconds
65% will be able to imitate a heel-toe walk
Many will have begun to throw overhand
Fine Motor:
Almost all will copy a circle and a + sign
80% will pick the longer line of two
50% will begin to draw a person in three parts
Language:
Speech is quite understandable in almost all
95% will give their first and last names
85% will understand cold, tired, hungry
80% will identify three of four colors

Psychosocial:
Almost all will play games with other children
70% will dress without supervision

Physical Examination (particular attention)

Update growth curves
Continued reassessment, search for new findings
Reminder that hearing and vision must be evaluated at each visit
Reminder that taking the blood pressure is an integral part of the physical examination

Anticipatory Guidance

Importance of reading to the child frequently
Need for a toddler car seat
Fears and fantasies
Separation (reliance on other adults as time goes by)
Safety (matches and lighters out of reach, strangers, the street, window guards)
Personal hygiene (again, the importance of frequent tooth-brushing)

Plans and Problems

Review immunizations and implement as appropriate
Consider the need for serum lead level, hemoglobin or hematocrit value, urinalysis
Maintain problem list, making appropriate plans, and, if necessary, referrals

5 Years of Age

History (interim details)

Parental concerns
Reassess social and system review

Development: By this age

Gross motor:
Almost all will hop nicely on one foot
75% will balance on one foot for as many as 10 seconds
60% will do a heel-toe walk backward reasonably well

Fine motor:
    85% will draw a person in three parts
    65% will draw a person in as many as 6 parts
    60% will copy a square
Language:
    Almost all will identify four colors
    Almost all will understand on, under, in front of, behind
    Well over half will define adequately five of the following eight words: ball, cake, desk, house, banana, curtain, fence, ceiling
Psychosocial:
    Almost all will dress without supervision
    Almost all will brush teeth without help
    Almost all will play board and card games
    Almost all will be relaxed when left with a babysitter
    More than half will prepare their own cereal

Physical Examination (particular attention)

Update growth curves
Continued reassessment, search for new findings

Anticipatory Guidance

Reading together
School readiness (plays with others, endures separation from parent[s])
Chores
Discipline (consistency, praising)
Sex identification, education
Peer interaction
Television
Safety (seat belts, guns, bike helmets, matches, swimming, memorize name, address, phone number)
(It is not usually possible to cover so many topics at one visit, so it is usually necessary to be selective based on your knowledge of the family situation.)

Plans and Problems

Review immunizations and implement as appropriate
Consider the need for a tuberculosis test, urinalysis
Maintain problem list, making appropriate plans and, if necessary, referrals

Elementary School Years (6 to 12 Years of Age)

History (interim details)

Parental concerns
Child's concerns
Reassess social and system review
    Attention span
    Behavior at home and in school
    School accomplishments and experience
    Enuresis, encopresis, constipation, nightmares

Development

By this time gross and fine motor problems have most often become apparent (but not always; the neurologic examination should not be shortchanged). Language and psychosocial skills can be readily investigated in talks with the parents and the child and in explorations of the school and play experiences. Socialization and developing maturity may have different expressions at home, on the playground, and in school, and in the variety of times with people of different ages and different degrees of acquaintance. Talks with teachers, report cards, and the various drawings and other efforts that the child brings home from school can be very helpful.

Physical Examination (particular attention)

Update growth curves
Continued reassessment, search for new findings
Begin Tanner stage assessment

Anticipatory Guidance

Parent-child rapport
Need for praise
Responsibility
Safety (seat belts, guns, fire, bike helmets, swimming, memorize name, address, phone number)
Allowance
Television
Sex education
Dental care
Adult supervision
Discipline (limit setting)

(Again, time constraints almost always make it necessary to adjust the menu for anticipatory guidance to your judgment about the family's needs.)

Plans and Problems

Review immunizations and implement as appropriate

Consider the need for a tuberculosis test, urinalysis

Maintain problem list, making appropriate plans and, if necessary, referrals

Adolescents

(Remember that we have assumed a continuing relationship with the patient from birth on; real life does not always allow that. If you are seeing a patient for the first time, you must, of course, begin with a full history and physical examination.)

History (interim details)

Patient's concerns

Parental concerns

Menstrual history

Use of tobacco, alcohol, street or other drugs

Diet and what guides it

Sexual activity (relationships, masturbation, pregnancy and disease control measures); the exact timing for all of this should rely on your assessment of the situation and your judgment; in general, the social experience

School experience

Suicidal ideation; be ever on the alert and bring it up when necessary

Update knowledge of home and social structure

Revisit in general social and system review

(An adolescent patient [and some elementary school children] may prefer to be or should be seen alone at times and, as they get older, most often or always. This does not mean, however, that the parents are not involved. The proper balance in this relies on your judgment.)

Development

By this time the adolescent's physical, neurologic, and cognitive abilities should be well understood, but nothing should be taken for granted. Conversation with the patient, parent(s), and school officials, school records, and, of course, a careful physical examination should all be helpful.

Physical Examination (particular attention)

Update growth curves
Continued reassessment, search for new findings
Tanner stage assessment
Spinal curvatures, particularly in early adolescent females

Anticipatory Guidance

Puberty and its issues; body image
Sexuality, sexually transmitted disease, contraception
Diet
Tobacco, alcohol, drugs
Risk-taking behavior
Exercise
Safety (guns, seat belts, bike helmets)
Family and other social relationships
Independence and responsibility
School and the future

(Time constraints almost always make it necessary to adjust the menu for anticipatory guidance to your judgment about the adolescent's and/or the family's needs.)

Plans and Problems

Review immunizations and implement as appropriate
Consider the need for tuberculosis test, sexually transmitted disease testing, hemoglobin or hematocrit determination, urinalysis, lipid screen
Maintain problem list, making appropriate plans and, if necessary, referrals

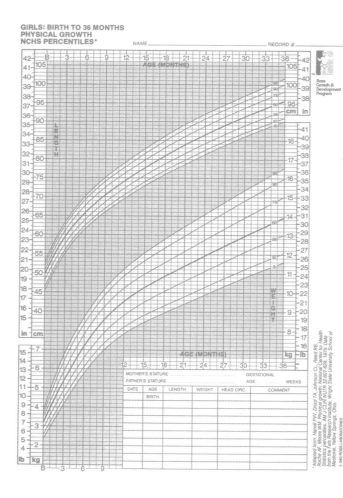

GIRLS: BIRTH TO 36 MONTHS
PHYSICAL GROWTH
NCHS PERCENTILES*

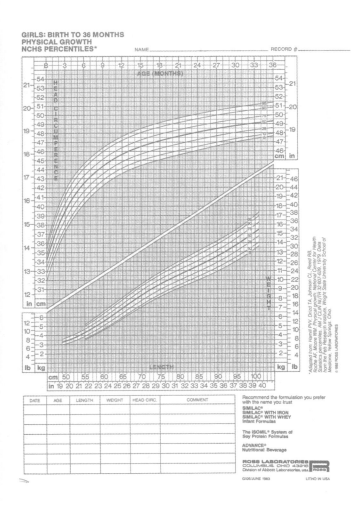

GIRLS: BIRTH TO 36 MONTHS
PHYSICAL GROWTH
NCHS PERCENTILES*

NAME _____   RECORD # _____

DATE	AGE	LENGTH	WEIGHT	HEAD CIRC.	COMMENT

Recommend the formulation you prefer
with the name you trust

SIMILAC®
SIMILAC® WITH IRON
SIMILAC® WITH WHEY
Infant Formulas

The ISOMIL® System of
Soy Protein Formulas

ADVANCE®
Nutritional Beverage

ROSS LABORATORIES
COLUMBUS, OHIO 43216
Division of Abbott Laboratories, USA

*Adapted from: Hamill PVV, Drizd TA, Johnson CL, Reed RB, Roche AF, Moore WM. Physical growth: National Center for Health Statistics percentiles. AM J CLIN NUTR 32:607-629, 1979. Data from the Fels Research Institute, Wright State University School of Medicine, Yellow Springs, Ohio.

© 1982 ROSS LABORATORIES

G105/JUNE 1983   LITHO IN USA

BOYS: BIRTH TO 36 MONTHS
PHYSICAL GROWTH
NCHS PERCENTILES*

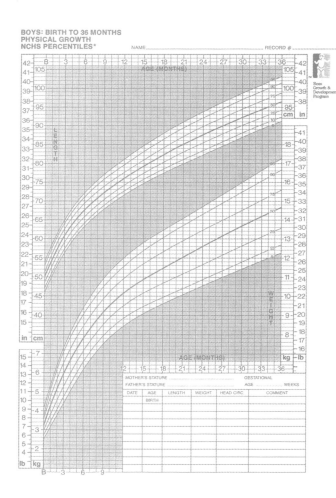

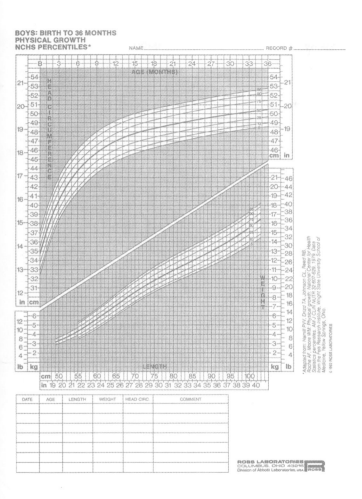

BOYS: BIRTH TO 36 MONTHS
PHYSICAL GROWTH
NCHS PERCENTILES*

NAME_____ RECORD #_____

DATE	AGE	LENGTH	WEIGHT	HEAD CIRC	COMMENT

GIRLS: 2 TO 18 YEARS
PHYSICAL GROWTH
NCHS PERCENTILES*

NAME _____ RECORD # _____

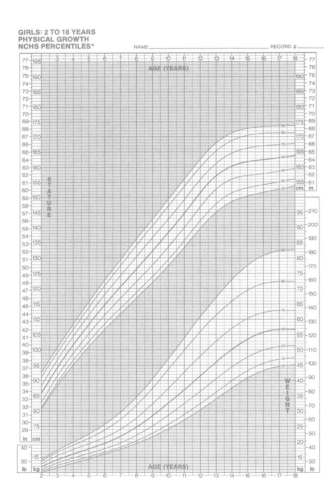

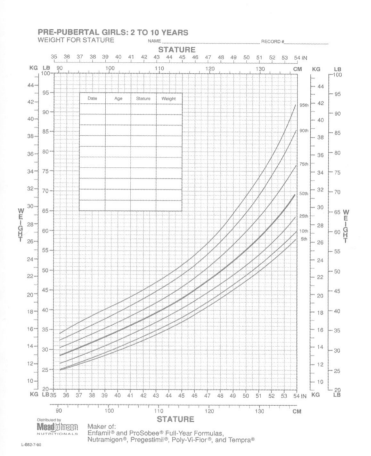

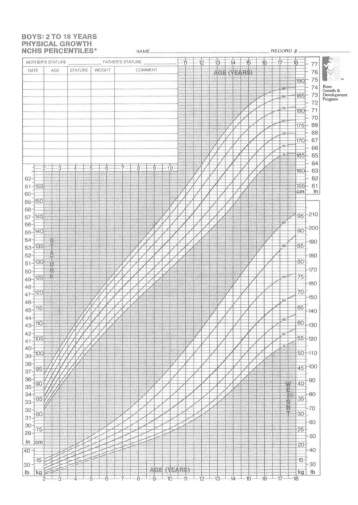

BOYS: 2 TO 18 YEARS
PHYSICAL GROWTH
NCHS PERCENTILES*

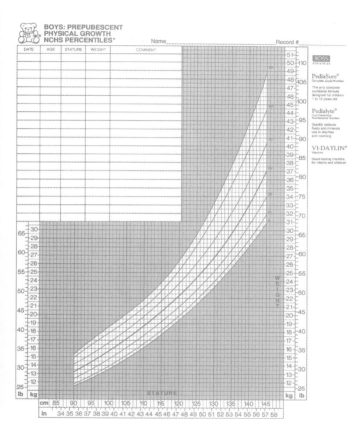

BOYS: PREPUBESCENT
PHYSICAL GROWTH
NCHS PERCENTILES*

SPECIAL CONSIDERATIONS FOR THE PREGNANT WOMAN

Use the same process of physical examination as for the adult.

In addition, perform more extensive abdominal and pelvic evaluations for pregnancy status and fetal well-being.

Late in pregnancy, a woman may find it difficult to assume the supine position without experiencing hypotension; use this position only when necessary.

Provide alternative positioning by elevating the backrest or by supplying pillows for the woman to assume the left side-lying position.

Have her empty her bladder to make the abdominal assessment more comfortable for her and more accurate.

Remember that during pregnancy, urinary urgency and frequency are common.

CHAPTER 21

REPORTING AND RECORDING

SUBJECTIVE DATA—THE HISTORY

Record the patient's history, especially in an initial visit, to provide a comprehensive data base. Arrange information appropriately in specific categories, usually in a particular sequence such as chronologic order with most recent information first. Include both positive and negative data that contribute to the assessment. Use the following organized sequence as a guide.

Identifying Information

Record the data recommended by the health agency.
   Patient's name
   Identification number/Social Security number
   Age, sex
   Marital status
   Address (home and business)
   Phone numbers
   Occupation, employer
   Insurance plan and number
   Date of visit
   For children and dependent adults, names of parents or next of kin
   Put identifying information on each page of record.

Source and Reliability of Information

   Document who is giving the history and the relationship to patient.
   Indicate when an old record is used.
   State judgment about the reliability of the information.

Chief Complaint

Description of the patient's main reason(s) for seeking health care, in patient's own words with quotation marks. Paraphrase only if this makes the complaint more clear.

Include the duration of the problem.

History of Present Problem

List and describe current symptoms of the chief complaint and their appearance chronologically in reverse order, dating events and symptoms.

List any expected symptoms that are absent.

Identify anyone in household with same symptoms.

Note pertinent information from the review of systems, family history, and personal/social history along with findings.

Where more than one problem is identified, address each in a separate paragraph, including the following details of symptom occurrence:

Onset: when the problem first started, setting and circumstances, manner of the onset (sudden versus gradual)

Location: exact location, localized or generalized, radiation patterns

Duration: how long problem has lasted, intermittent or continuous, duration of each episode

Character: nature of symptom

Aggravating/associated factors: food, activity, rest, certain movements; nausea, vomiting, diarrhea, fever, chills, etc.

Relieving factors: prescribed and/or self-remedies, their effect on the problem; food, rest, heat, ice, activity, position, etc.

Temporal factors: frequency; relation to other symptoms, problems, functions; sequence of events

Severity of the symptoms: quantify on a 0 to 10 scale; effect on the patient's life-style

Medical History

List and describe each of the following with dates of occurrence and any specific information available:

General health and strength over lifetime as patient perceives it

Hospitalization and/or surgery: dates, hospital, diagnosis, complications

Injuries and disabilities

Major childhood illnesses

Adult illnesses

Immunizations: polio, diphtheria-pertussis-tetanus, tetanus toxoid, influenza, cholera, typhus, typhoid, bacille Calmette-

Guérin (BCG), last purified protein derivative (PPD) or other skin tests, unusual reaction to immunizations

Medications: past, current, and recent medications (prescribed, nonprescription, home remedies), dosages

Allergies: drugs, foods, environmental

Transfusions: reason, date, and number of units transfused, reactions

Emotional status: history of mood disorders, psychiatric attention or medications

Family History

Present information about the age and health of family members in narrative or genogram form, including at least three generations.

Family members: include parents, grandparents, aunts and uncles, siblings, spouse, and children. For deceased family members, note the age at time of death and cause, if known.

Major health or genetic disorders: include hypertension, cancer, cardiac, respiratory, renal, cerebrovascular or thyroid disorders, asthma or other allergic manifestations, blood dyscrasias, psychiatric difficulties, tuberculosis, diabetes mellitus, hepatitis, or other familial disorders.

Personal/Social History

Include information according to the concerns of the patient and the influence of the health problem on the patient's and family's life:

Cultural background and practices, birthplace, position in family

Marital status

Religious preference, religious proscriptions for medical care

Education; economic condition, housing, number in household

Occupation: work conditions and hours, physical or mental strain, protective devices used; exposure to chemicals, toxins, poisons, fumes, smoke, asbestos, or radioactive material at home or work

Environment: home, school, work; structural barriers if handicapped, community services utilized; travel; exposure to contagious diseases

Current health habits and/or risk factors: exercise, smoking, salt intake, weight control; diet, vitamins and other supplements, caffeine-containing beverages; alcohol or recreational drug use; response to CAGE questions related to alcohol use; participation in a drug or alcohol treatment program or support group

General life satisfaction, hobbies, interests, sources of stress

Review of Systems

Organize in a general head-to-toe sequence, including an impression of each symptom.

Record expected or negative findings as the absence of symptoms or problems.

When unexpected or positive findings are stated by the patient, include details from further inquiry as you would in the present illness.

Include the following categories of information (sequence may vary):

General constitutional symptoms
Diet
Skin, hair, and nails
Head and neck
Eyes, ears, nose, mouth, and throat
Endocrine
Breasts
Heart and blood vessels
Chest and lungs
Hematologic
Lymphatic
Immunologic
Gastrointestinal
Genitourinary
Musculoskeletal
Neurologic
Psychiatric

PHYSICAL FINDINGS

General Statement

Age, race, sex, general appearance
Nutritional status, weight, height, and frame size

Vital signs: temperature, pulse rate, respiratory rate, blood pressure (two extremities, two positions)

Mental Status

Physical appearance and behavior
Memory, reasoning, attention span, response to questions
Mental status exam score
Voice quality, articulation, content, coherence, comprehension
Anxiety, disturbance in thought content

Skin

Color, integrity, temperature, hydration, tattoos
Presence of edema, excessive perspiration, unusual odor
Presence and description of lesions (size, shape, location, inflammation, tenderness, induration, discharge), parasites
Hair texture and distribution
Nail configuration, color, texture, condition, presence of clubbing, nail plate adherence, firmness

Head

Size and contour of head, scalp appearance and movement
Facial features (characteristics, symmetry)
Presence of edema or puffiness, tenderness
Temporal arteries: characteristics

Eyes

Visual acuity, visual fields
Appearance of orbits, conjunctivae, sclerae, eyelids, eyebrows
Pupillary shape, consensual response to light and accommodation, extraocular movements, corneal light reflex, cover-uncover test
Ophthalmoscopic findings of cornea, lens, retina, optic disc, macula, retinal vessel size, caliber and arteriovenous crossings

Ears

Configuration, position and alignment of auricles
Otoscopic findings of canals (cerumen, lesions, discharge, foreign body) and tympanic membranes (integrity, color, landmarks, mobility, perforation)
Hearing: air and bone conduction tests, whispered voice

Nose

Appearance of external nose, nasal patency, flaring

Nasal mucosa and septum, color, alignment, discharge, crusting, polyp

Appearance of turbinates

Presence of sinus tenderness or swelling

Discrimination of odors

Mouth and Throat

Number, occlusion and condition of teeth; presence of dental appliances

Lips, tongue, buccal and oral mucosa, and floor of mouth (color, moisture, surface characteristics, ulcerations, induration, symmetry)

Oropharynx, tonsils, palate (color, symmetry, exudate)

Symmetry and movement of tongue, soft palate and uvula; gag reflex

Discrimination of taste

Neck

Mobility, suppleness, and strength

Position of trachea

Thyroid size, shape, tenderness, and nodules

Presence of masses, webbing, skinfolds

Chest

Size and shape of chest, anteroposterior versus transverse diameter, symmetry of movement with respiration

Presence of retractions, use of accessory muscles

Lungs

Respiratory rate, depth, regularity, quietness or ease of respiration

Palpation findings: symmetry and quality of tactile fremitus, thoracic expansion

Percussion findings: quality and symmetry of percussion notes, diaphragmatic excursion

Auscultation findings: characteristics of breath sounds (pitch, duration, intensity, vesicular, bronchial, bronchovesicular) unexpected breath sounds

Characteristics of cough

Presence of friction rub, egophony, whispered pectoriloquy or bronchophony

Breasts

Size, contour

Symmetry, texture, masses, scars, tenderness, thickening, nodules, discharge, retraction, or dimpling

Characteristics of nipples and areolae

Heart

Anatomic location of apical impulse

Heart rate, rhythm, amplitude, contour, and symmetry of apical impulse

Palpation findings: pulsations, thrills, heaves, or lifts

Auscultation findings: characteristics of S_1 and S_2 (location, intensity, pitch, timing, splitting, systole, diastole)

Presence of murmurs, clicks, snaps, S_3 or S_4 (timing, location, radiation intensity, pitch, quality)

Blood Vessels

Blood pressure: comparison between extremities, with position change

Jugular vein pulsations and distention, pressure measurement

Presence of bruits over carotid, temporal, renal, and femoral arteries, abdominal aorta

Pulses in distal extremities

Temperature, color, hair distribution, skin texture, nail beds of lower extremities

Presence of edema, swelling, vein distention, Homan sign, or tenderness of lower extremities

Abdomen

Shape, contour, visible aorta pulsations, venous patterns, hernia

Auscultation findings: bowel sounds in all quadrants, their character

Palpation findings: aorta, organs, feces, masses, location, size, contour, consistency, tenderness, muscle resistance

Percussion findings: areas of different percussion notes, costovertebral angle tenderness

Liver span

Male Genitalia

Appearance of external genitalia, circumcision status, location and size of urethral opening, smegma discharge, lesions, distribution of pubic hair

Palpation findings: penis, testes, epididymides, vas deferens, contour, consistency, tenderness

Presence of hernia or scrotal swelling

Female Genitalia

Appearance of external genitalia and perineum, distribution of pubic hair, inflammation, excoriation, tenderness, scarring, discharge

Internal examination findings: appearance of vaginal mucosa, cervix, discharge, odor, lesions

Bimanual examination findings: size, position, tenderness of cervix, vaginal walls, uterus, adnexae, and ovaries

Rectovaginal examination findings

Urinary incontinence with bearing down

Anus and Rectum

Sphincter control, presence of hemorrhoids, fissures, skin tags, polyps

Rectal wall contour, tenderness, sphincter tone

Prostate size, contour, consistency, mobility

Color and consistency of stool

Lymphatic

Presence of lymph nodes in neck, epitrochlear, axillary, or inguinal areas

Size, shape, consistency, warmth, tenderness, mobility, discreteness of nodes

Musculoskeletal

Posture: alignment of extremities and spine, symmetry of body parts

Symmetry of muscle mass, tone and strength; grading of strength, fasciculations, spasms

Range of motion, passive and active; presence of pain with movement

Appearance of joints; presence of deformities, tenderness or crepitus

Neurologic

Cranial nerves: specific findings for each or specify those tested, if findings are recorded in head and neck sections

Cerebellar and motor function: gait, balance, coordination with rapid alternating motions

Sensory function, symmetry (touch, pain, vibration, temperature, monofilament)

Superficial and deep tendon reflexes: symmetry, grade

ASSESSMENT

Diagnoses with rationale, based on subjective and objective data

Anticipated potential problems

Disease progression or complication

New problem

PLAN

Diagnostic tests ordered or performed

Therapeutic treatment plan

Patient education

Referrals initiated

Future visit to evaluate plan

REFERENCES

Barkauskas VH et al: *Health and physical assessment,* ed 2, St Louis, 1998, Mosby.

Edge V, Miller M: *Women's health care,* St Louis, 1994, Mosby.

Farrar WE et al: *Infectious diseases,* ed 2, London, 1992, Gower.

Folstein M et al: The meaning of cognitive impairment in the elderly, *J Am Geriatr Soc* 33(4):228, 1985.

Frisancho AR: New norms of upper limb fat and muscle areas for assessment of nutritional status, *Am J Clin Nutr* 34:2540, 1981.

Goldman MP, Fitzpatrick RE: *Cutaneous laser surgery: the art and science of selective photothermolysis,* 1994, Mosby.

Habif TP: *Clinical dermatology,* ed 3, St Louis, 1996, Mosby.

Harvey AM et al: *The principles and practice of medicine,* ed 22, Chapters 2, 7, p. 91, Table 2. 7-2, Norwalk Conn/San Mateo, Calif, 1988, Appleton & Lange.

Judge R et al: *Clinical diagnosis,* ed 5, Boston, 1988 Little, Brown.

Koop CE: The Surgeon General's letter on child sexual abuse, *US DHHS,* 1988.

McCarty DJ: *Arthritis and allied conditions: a textbook of rheumatology,* ed 2, Philadelphia, 1993, Lea & Febiger.

Miyasaki-Ching CM: *Chasteen's essentials of clinical dental assisting,* ed 5, St Louis, 1997, Mosby.

National Institutes of Health: second report of the Expert Panel on Detection, Evaluation, and Treatment of High Blood Cholesterol in Adults, National Institutes of Health No. 93-3096, Washington, DC, September 1993, National Institutes of Health.

National Institutes of Health No. 48-4080, November 1997.

Samiy AH et al: *Textbook of diagnostic medicine,* p. 190, Table 7-3, Philadelphia, 1987, Lea & Febiger.

Seidel HM et al: *Mosby's guide to physical examination,* ed 4, St Louis, 1999, Mosby.

Smith RD, McNamara JJ (1984): The neurologic examination in children with school problems, *J of School Health,* 54(7): 231-234, 1984.

Thomas AE et al: A nomogram method for assessing body weight, *Am J Clin Nutr* 29(3):302-304, 1976

Thompson JM et al: *Clinical nursing,* ed 4, St Louis, 1997, Mosby.

Thompson JM, Wilson SF: *Health assessment for nursing practice,* 1996, Mosby.

Update on task force report on high blood pressure in children, *Pediatrics* 98:649, 1996.

U.S. Department of Health and Human Services: *Clinician's handbook of preventive services,* Washington, DC, 1994, U.S. Government Printing Office.

U.S. Preventive Services Task Force: *Guide to clinical preventive services,* ed 2, Washington, DC, 1996, U.S. Government Printing Office.

Weston WL, Lane AT, Morelli JG: *Color textbook of pediatric dermatology,* ed 2, St Louis, 1996, Mosby.

White GM: *Color atlas of regional dermatology,* St Louis, 1994, Mosby.

Zitelli BJ, Davis HW: *Atlas of pediatric physical diagnosis,* ed 3, St Louis, 1997, Mosby.

Index

CLINICAL AND
REFERENCE NOTES

CLINICAL AND
REFERENCE NOTES

CLINICAL AND
REFERENCE NOTES

CLINICAL AND
REFERENCE NOTES

CLINICAL AND
REFERENCE NOTES